Serenella Besio, Daniela Bulgarelli and Vaska Stancheva-Popkostadinova (Eds.)
Play development in children with disabilities

Serenella Besio, Daniela Bulgarelli
and Vaska Stancheva-Popkostadinova (Eds.)

Play development in children with disabilities

DE GRUYTER
OPEN

ISBN 978-3-11-052211-2
e-ISBN (PDF) 978-3-11-052214-3
e-ISBN (EPUB) 978-3-11-052219-8

Published by De Gruyter Open Ltd, Warsaw/Berlin
Part of Walter de Gruyter GmbH, Berlin/Boston
The book is published with open access at www.degruyter.com.

Library of Congress Cataloging-in-Publication Data
A CIP catalog record for this book has been applied for at the Library of Congress.

www.degruyteropen.com
Cover illustration: Enzo Sanny (8 years), Italy

Contents

Acknowledgements

We would like to warmly thank the LUDI reviewers of the whole text, Angharad Beckett and Rianne Jansens: their contribution has been precious. A particular thank also to Anna Andreeva, Francesca Caprino, Sylvie Ray, Hilary Gardner, Odile Perino, and Mira Tzvetkova-Arsova for their competent and careful reciprocal revision of the chapters.

Serenella Besio, Daniela Bulgarelli,
and Vaska Stancheva-Popkostadinova

Introduction

Why Play and Which Play for Children with Disabilities?

Article 31 of the Convention on the Rights of the Child (United Nations, 1989) grants the child the right to rest and leisure, be able to engage in play and recreational activities appropriate to the age of the child, and participate freely in cultural life and the arts.[1]

The same Convention also pursues the right to social inclusion, intended as a general framework for democratic societies, and as a model of intervention that promotes everyone's participation, respecting possibilities and constraints, cultural stories and differences.

Every nation is currently involved in the efforts towards general inclusion in societies, particularly with regards to education and training institutions and to legislative systems. This may result in further deprivation, given the importance of social sharing in peer play: in this sense, the inclusion of children with disabilities remains an unreached goal.

But these children have the right to play, and without it, they have limited chances for development. The Convention of the Rights of Persons with Disabilities (United Nations, 2006) recognises this risk and dedicates Article 7 to the expression and protection of the rights of children with disabilities, emphasising the need to guarantee them proper educational process in an inclusive and life-long educational system (Art. 24), as well as the right to participate in recreational activities, sports, and entertainment, including those that take place in schools (Art. 30).

It can then be stated that play is widely recognised as the fundamental activity for the overall development of every child. It drives a major role in the acquisition of cognitive, socio-psychological, and relational skills, but it is also an innate 'engine' for curiosity, challenge, motivation towards action, and social relationships.

Play is spontaneous and voluntary, and it has no extrinsic goals: it is never lazy, while on the contrary, it requires concentration, intensity, and it produces enjoyment and fun.

---

1 This paragraph of the *Introduction* and partially the second one are highly inspired to: 1) Besio, S., & Carnesecchi, M. (2011). *Memorandum of Understanding of the COST Action "LUDI. Play for Children with Disabilities"*. COST Association, Bruxelles, retrieved from: http://w3.cost.eu/fileadmin/domain_files/TDP/Action_TD1309/mou/TD1309-e.pdf; 2) Besio, S., Carnesecchi, M., & Encarnação, P. (2015). Introducing LUDI: a Research Network on Play for Children with Disabilities. *Studies in Health Technology and Informatics*. 217:689-95.

Children with disabilities may be deprived from playing as a direct consequence of their impairments and/or because the environment is not adequate enough or suitably accommodated, so that they can have access to forms and contexts of play in which they can take part.

The scientific core issue adopted by LUDI, as the following figure shows, lies at the crossroads of three autonomous research areas: disability (impairments' types, functioning characteristics), play (play characterisation and development, play assessment, right to play), and environmental factors (technology, contexts, play situations and scenarios).

These three areas also reflect the main domains of the International Classification of Functioning, Disability and Health promoted by the World Health Organisation in 2001,[2] which enables to describe the human functioning in relation to the activity and the participation and with respect to the contextual aspects of daily life, in particular, environmental and personal factors.

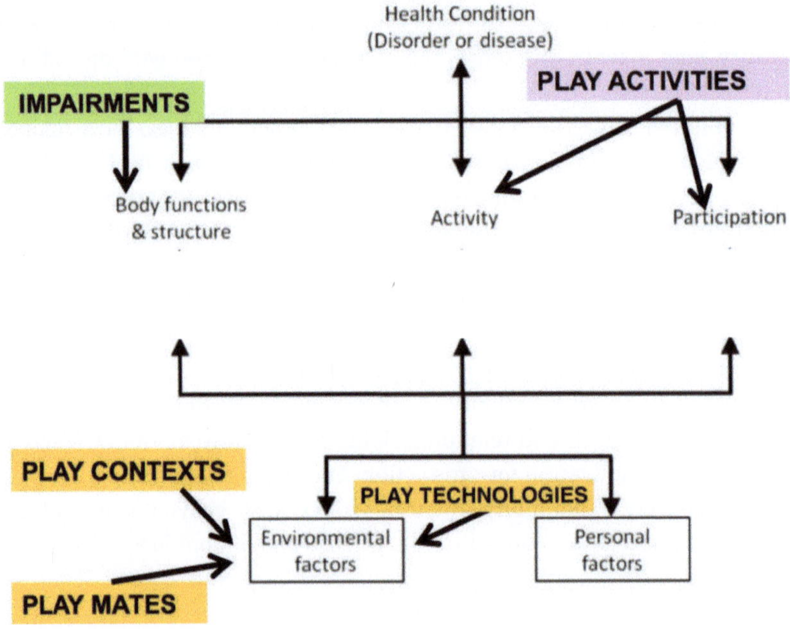

Figure 1. Factors involving children with disabilities' play activity (Besio, Carnesecchi, & Encarnaç*ão*, *2015*)

2 *International Classification of Functioning, Disability and Health*—ICF (WHO, 2001). The version for Children and Youth (ICF-CY) has been delivered in 2009.

A large collection of studies of excellence has been devoted in the last decades, in different countries, to the topic of play for children with disabilities. Anyway, they have been mostly confined to specific niches, without exploring these areas of research from a fully interdisciplinary perspective; for example, they have included: development of social robotic tools, implementation of adapted toys, or creation of new accessible playgrounds; creation of new tools of evaluation for specific impairments; studies in the field of design.

Those initiatives, however, still lack a common systematisation, thus making play for children with disabilities a not yet recognised area of research; furthermore, in almost all these areas of study, these children's play is viewed only as the mean through which they can accomplish clinical and therapeutic goals. The extrinsic goal of these educational and rehabilitation projects is mainly the functional recovery of impairments; they should be considered more as 'play-like' activities, rather than truly play activities *per se*: in other words, children are not engaged purely for the sake of play.

To grant children with disabilities the full exercise of their right to play means to focus on the engagement connected with ludic activities as an end rather than as a mean. By taking into account 'play for play's sake' activities, the purpose of LUDI is to create general awareness on their impact in the quality of life of children with disabilities, and to initiate a process of cultural and social change that will break down the barriers that hinder the full exercise of their right to play and the realisation of a true social inclusion.

The COST Action 'LUDI—Play for Children with Disabilities' and its Challenges

'LUDI—Play for Children with Disabilities' is an Action (2014-2018) financed by COST (European Cooperation Science and Technology); it is a multidisciplinary network including now 32 countries and almost 100 researchers and practitioners belonging to the humanistic and technological fields, aimed at studying the topic of play for children with disabilities.[3]

The LUDI Action has the primary objective of spreading awareness of the importance of providing children with disabilities the opportunity to play. Given the importance of play for child development, the Action stems from the belief that it is necessary to ensure an equal right to play and to put play at the centre of both multidisciplinary research and intervention practices directed at children with disabilities. The LUDI network is organised into four Working Groups (WGs):

- WG1: Children's play in relation to the types of disabilities
- WG2: Technology for the play of children with disabilities

3 The Action websites are the following ones: www.cost.eu/TD1309; www.ludi-network.eu.

- WG3: Contexts for the play of children with disabilities
- WG4: Methods, technology, and frameworks for the development of the child with disabilities' play

WG1 provides the Action framework, including operational definitions of the main concepts around play and disability. WG2 compiles and distils the existing knowledge on technology to support play for children with disabilities. WG3 analyses the different contexts of play and identifies current barriers hindering children with disabilities the right to play. Finally, WG4 builds on the work of all the other WGs and proposes methods, technologies, and frameworks to support play for children with disabilities.

To accomplish its objectives, the LUDI Action will carry out three main tasks: a) collecting and systematising all existing competence and skills: educational research, clinical initiatives, and using the know-how of resources centres and users' associations; b) developing new knowledge related to settings, technology (devices, services, strategies, and practices) associated with the play of children with disabilities; and c) disseminating the best practices emerging from the joint effort of researchers, practitioners, and users.

The LUDI network is entrusted with a really ambitious and ground-breaking goal, branching into many prospects of exploration and susceptible to significant developments in several fields. New knowledge is expected in all the scientific-related areas, not only in the 'speciality' of disability, but as overall acquisitions about play (development, tools, relationships, activities, human rights, and so on) and child development.

This new knowledge will creatively nurture, in its turn, the fields of technological and tool development, clinical and engineering research, education and rehabilitation practice. A more stable and consistent awareness on the child's play development would give more suitable frameworks to professionals and researchers to make their interventions and proposals more effective. A more widespread sensibleness on the social aspects and value of play would result in disseminating inclusive contexts and methods.

At the same time, a shared belief on the importance of play—for the sake of play—for children with disabilities as for any other child, as well as on the role of inclusion for the upcoming human societies, will demand changes in many aspects of cultural and social life: to make only some examples, the accessibility of the mainstream play sites and tools, the concrete application of the right to play for every child, the adoption of a new mindset on disability, less focused on recovery and more interested in childhood's fundamentals.

The main challenge is already inside the network, which is both international and multi-disciplinary. Researchers and professionals who belong to LUDI come, in fact, from many European countries, bringing with them their social and cultural beliefs and experiences, which should be explored and compared, and are expert in different fields, which should be merged together through deep and patent discussion. The purpose of this massive mediation activity is to reach reciprocal understanding and to develop new common, collective wisdom, in the light of the basic statements shared since the beginning of the work.

But this is an extensive process, as shifting to new paradigms always requires a long time and a lot of determination.[4] This means, for example, that at the initial life of LUDI, in its first publications—as this one is—some incoherence still exists between authors and proposed approaches, and that the debate is currently open and active. Any product of LUDI is then a part of a recursive process, whose results should be considered, until its end, as partial steps of a long road.

The Purpose of this Book

This book is the first deliverable of the WG1 'Children's play in relation to the types of disabilities', part of the LUDI network. As already said, WG1 is devoted to the topics of definition of play, classification of impairments accordingly to DSM-5 and ICD-10, and classifications of types of play with respect to the cognitive complexity, and the degree and type of social interaction. This book is the result of the first two-year of activities of WG1.

The main objective of this book is to bring the LUDI contribution to the important topic of play and children with disabilities, because an international consensus on these two areas is still lacking in the related literature and also in the overall practice. In particular, there is not a shared and general agreement on a clear definition of play and play activities, especially when they are related to children with some kind of impairments, and/or when ludic contexts accessible for these children are drawn up.

Three steps should be achieved to support the right to play of children with disabilities, ensure equity in its exercise, and spread awareness on the importance of giving them the opportunity to play: first, adopt a 'common language', at least all over Europe; second, to put play at the centre of the multidisciplinary research and intervention regarding the children with disabilities; third, to grant this topic the status of a scientific and social theme of full visibility and recognised authority.

In fact, children with disabilities face several limitations in play: they might not be able to play; might not want to play; might not know how to play; might not recognise a situation or a object for their ludic characteristics; they can isolate themselves from the others' play; might be scared by a play situation; might prefer to repeat the same play, in the same way, in the same site.

4 We thank Dr. Ute Navidi, who served as first reviewer for the LUDI activities, commissioned by COST, for this very encouraging statement, that we immediately incorporated in our vision.

These limitations can be due to several reasons: impairments to body functions and structures can impede or make some actions and activities very difficult; playgrounds, toys, and other play tools can prove not to be accessible and usable; social and built environments and contexts may be neither accessible nor inclusive. Furthermore, the world of the adults around these children might show several lacks: in educational awareness and intentionality; in specific psycho-pedagogical and rehabilitative competence; in effective intervention methodologies. Moreover, these children's lives are dominated by medical and rehabilitative practices, in which play is always considered as an ancillary but very fruitful activity able to reach an instrumental objective or to pursue an improvement.

Play for the sake of play is considered, mainly for children with disabilities, a waste of time.

The concept of play for the sake of play strongly refers to the distinction between 'play' and 'play-like' activities. Play activities are initiated and carried out by the player (alone, with peers, with adults, and so on) only for the purpose of play itself (fun and joy, interest and challenge, love of race and competition, ilinx and dizziness, and so on). They have of course consequences on growth and development, but these consequences are not intentionally pursued. Play-like activities are initiated and conducted by an adult (with one or more children), in educational, clinical, social contexts; they are playful and pleasant, but their main objective is other than play: for example, cognitive learning, social learning, functional rehabilitation, child's observation and assessment, psychological support, psychotherapy. This book would intend to contribute to make a clear distinction between play and play-like activities that, hopefully, will bring to new developments in play studies.

Organisation of the Contents

This book sets itself as the basis for the further work of the COST Action 'LUDI—Play for Children with Disabilities', by establishing some important cornerstones, after a careful overview of the literature existing in the related fields. Its contents are organised as follows:

- Chapter 1 presents the theme of children's play in its countless facets, with special reference to 'The need of play for the sake of play' (Serenella Besio).
- Chapter 2 deals with one of its special characteristics, the fact that play should be considered a child's right, also in the case of disability: 'The right of Children with Disabilities to play' (Keith Towler, from the International Play Association—IPA).
- Chapters 3 and 4 are, respectively, focused on the 'Conceptual review of play' and 'Conceptual review of disabilities'; they take into account the existing definitions of these two crucial constructs as well as the major scientific classifications existing in the international literature, and finally, propose the

LUDI Classifications of play and of disability to be adopted (Nicole Bianquin and Daniela Bulgarelli).

- Chapters 5 to 11 deepen the characteristics that play might assume in case of different types of impairments, according to the LUDI Classification; the authors of each chapters tried to take into account the aspects of play for the sake of play, as far as possible with reference to the existing literature. In particular, they are the following ones:
  - Play in children with intellectual disabilities (Daniela Bulgarelli and Vaska Stancheva-Popkostadinova)
  - Play in children with hearing impairments (Anna Andreeva, Pietro Celo, Nicole Vian)
  - Play in children with visual impairments (Mira Tzvetkova-Arsova and Tamara Zappaterra)
  - Play in children with communication disorders (Vardit Kindler and Natalia Amelina)
  - Play in children with physical impairments (Serenella Besio and Natalia Amelina)
  - Play in children with Autism Spectrum Disorders (Sylvie Ray-Kaeser, Evelyne Thommen, Laetitia Baggioni, and Miodrag Stanković)
  - Play in children with multiple disabilities (Francesca Caprino and Vittoria Stucci)
- Then, three chapters follow, which discuss about the contributions of different fields of research and clinical intervention to the promotion of play for the sake of play.
  - Chapter 12 reports the experiences from occupational therapy: The contribution of occupational therapy perspective to the promotion of play for the sake of play (Sylvie Ray-Kaeser and Helen Lynch).
  - Chapter 13 concerns the special pedagogy perspective: The contribution of special education to the promotion of play for the sake of play (Michele Mainardi).
  - Chapter 14 faces the theme of early intervention: Play for Early Intervention for children with disabilities (Vaska Stancheva-Popkostadinova and Tatjana Zorcec).
- Chapter 15—Mainstream toys for play—is related to an overview of mainstream toys, accompanied by some hints to single out their characteristics with respect to the different types of impairments, but also to the different types of toys (Odile Perino and Serenella Besio). It is not intended to be exhaustive of the issue ‘tools for playing’, but it wants to propose a first framework to interpret the world of commercial toys and to learn how to navigate inside, from the perspective of a generic adult, like, for example, a parent.
- The final and last Chapter 16 devises some reflections about the environmental barriers that can be found in the environment to establish interesting and

playful activities for children with disabilities—Influence of Environmental Factors on Play for Children with Disabilities–an overview. As this chapter is contemporarily an excerpt and a reworking of a publication that has been completed by members of LUDI WG3, the authors of this chapter are the same of that publication (Angharad Beckett, Carol Barron, Nan Cannon Jones, Marieke Coussens, Annemie Desoete, Helen Lynch, Maria Prellwitz, Deborah Fenney Salkeld).[5]

5 Barron, C., Beckett, A. E., Cannon-Jones, N., Coussens, M., Desoete, A., Fenney, D., Lynch, H., & Prellwitz, M. (*Forthcoming*). *Barriers to play and recreation for children with disabilities*. Berlin, D: De Gruyter.

Serenella Besio

1 The Need for Play for the Sake of Play

Put more simply, play as we know it is primarily a fortification against the disabilities of life
Brian Sutton-Smith

1.1 Defining Play[1]

> "I believed that, when most of [the] scholars talked about play, they fundamentally presupposed it to be either a form of progress, an exercise in power, a reliance on fate, a claim for identity, a form of frivolity, an issue of the imagination, or a manifestation of personal experience. My argument held that play was ambiguous, and the evidence for that ambiguity lay in these quite different scholarly ways of viewing play. Further, over the years it became clear to me that much of play was by itself—in its very nature, we might say—intentionally ambiguous (as, for example, is teasing) regardless of [...] general cultural frames" (Sutton-Smith, 2008:112).

So, what is play, then? It is seriousness and frivolity: reality and make-believe: rules and freedom. Within these antinomies lies the human experience of play, which must cope with a frustrating dichotomy that is always resolved through action. This duality is so deeply rooted in the phenomenon of play that Sutton-Smith based his last 'theory of play' on it—called 'coevolutionary multiplex of functions'—where play is described along five adaptive layers of 'dualudics'.

Rivers of ink have been spilled in an attempt to find a universally accepted definition of play, especially in different cultural environments. A now old but fascinating definition is provided by Fink: "Play resembles an oasis of happiness that we happen upon in the desert of our Tantalus-like seeking and pursuit of happiness. We are abducted by play. By playing we are released a bit from the mechanism of life—as if we were transported to another celestial body, where life appears easier, more ethereal, happier" (Fink, 1986).[2]

1 For the purpose of this chapter, it is important to stress here again that, within the LUDI framework, for children with disabilities, play has the same meaning and the same value that it has for all the children. This fact has one main consequence: all discourse surrounding play and children with disabilities must derive from and be strictly connected to the discourse concerning play in general. For this reason, the reflection on play here is developed from the overall immeasurable literature on play.
2 This paragraph has been inspired by Besio (2008).

Since ancient Greece, play has been recognised as a peculiar activity of the human being, at any age.[3] According to Aristotle, it should be distinguished from work, because it lacks necessity, and like virtue and happiness, it is rather characterised by freedom and self-sufficiency. Centuries later, Kant associated it to an aesthetic condition, because it is able to make imagination and intellect act together.

But since it began to be studied and analysed in an effort to recognise and understand it, play escaped any definition that tried to fix it, define it, encode it.

A fundamental attempt to find a comprehensive definition of play is offered by Huizinga in his famous book *Homo Ludens*, where it is described as the driving force of all human activities, a sort of primordial big bang from which civilisation itself comes from: "culture arises in the form of play, [...] it is played from the very beginning" (1967:46). While fulfilling the physiological and biological functions, according to the author, play can be defined as "a free activity standing quite consciously outside 'ordinary' life as being 'not serious', but at the same time absorbing the player intensely and utterly. It is an activity connected with no material interest, and no profit can be gained by it. It proceeds within its own proper boundaries of time and space according to fixed rules and in an orderly manner. It promotes the formation of social groupings which tend to surround themselves with secrecy and to stress their difference from the common world by disguise or other means" (1967:13).

In literature, from the educational, psychological and legal fields,[4] different and overlapping definitions have been proposed that focus attention on certain aspects.

Each of them gives a sense of fulfilment and seems both to compensate for a lack of interpretation and to underline an absence. After all, as stated by Bondioli (2002), each of these models seems only to reduce a huge theme to one of its small and basically limited aspects.

In short, play is indefinably play, to the point that Miller (1973) proposes to abandon the challenge of finding a single definition. In front of the baboon cage at the

---

3 Play, according to Gily, "is not a right for only a few men, if anything younger people, but it is a necessity for all. It interprets taking action according to spontaneity, originality, and the free exercise of one's faculties. Depressed by prolonged labor, the play instinct remains on the edges of ordinary human life, but emerges as soon as ease and hope liberate a space for its insurmountable need, such an obvious and recognizable need that man did not lose time to explain or to deify it. Its meaning is so clear that it does not require arguments, so urgent to overcome poverty and sadness: it has only end in itself, it justifies by itself" (2006:16).

4 The International Play Association Declaration on the child's rights to play maintains that "play is an essential part of childhood. All children have a right to experience play which, in the words of the Declaration, is free, open, boundless, sometimes chaotic, sometimes transformative. Play is a right which all adults have a responsibility to uphold. [...] The IPA Declaration highlights the growing evidence of the effects of lack of time and space for play and the serious and life-long effects on children's bodies and minds. IPA wishes to alert the wider community to this evidence and call for action to address this deprivation before the effects cause lifelong damage to more children". Theresa Casey, President, IPA, http://www.ipaworld.org.

zoo, people know—and there is general agreement on it—if the animals are playing, but they cannot explain why, and on what criteria they base their assertion. Similarly, Bundy (1993; 2000), who introduced an interesting *test of playfulness*,[5] concludes: "everyone knows whether a child or some children are playing. That is play: what is recognized as such by common observers".

To develop its project, the COST Action LUDI—Play for Children with Disabilities chose to adopt the definition proposed by Garvey: "Play is a range of voluntary, intrinsically motivated activities normally associated with recreational pleasure and enjoyment" (1990:4).

Even if the identification of a definition establishes an important point of agreement and sharing for researchers in the network, this is not enough, for the same reasons discussed earlier, to exhaust the discussion on the theme of play.

In what follows, some in-depth proposals are presented on certain aspects of play that have been considered important to study this phenomenon and its development in children with various types of impairments: in particular, the characteristics of play, its fundamentals, and the main functions it accomplishes.

It is believed that these elements can be useful for analysing, on the one hand, the difficulties that children with disabilities may encounter in their play activities and, on the other, the specific consequences that any deprivation of fun activities may cause to their development as a whole.

1.2 Play Characteristics

There are numerous proposals of 'essential traits' or 'characteristics' of play in literature in this field. According to Bateson (1956), they can be summarised in: *unfinalisation, creativity, not literalness, flexibility, pleasure.* Levy's proposal (1978) includes the following three traits: *intrinsic motivation* (motivation for the activity for the sake of the activity itself), *suspension of reality* (putting reality aside), and *internal locus of control* (the child has self-control); and Lillemyr (2009) adds *interactions in play.*

Within LUDI, play characteristics are the distinctive qualities of play, common to all its types, which contribute to giving the phenomenon its special peculiarity; only some proposals—among those highlighted by the various authors who have studied play—are presented as follows: they have been chosen as important elements of attention, harbingers of reflections and developments when it comes to play and children with disabilities. These qualities, shortly described in what follows, are: the feeling of *freedom*, its association with *concentration* and *intensity* (rather than with laziness), as well as with *pleasure* and/or with *fun*; in addition, the fact that

5 See also Bundy et al. (2001); Meakins et al. (2005).

play is always conducted in *serious* ways, driven by *curiosity* and *surprise*, *intrinsic motivation*, and finally, by *challenge*.

The first feature that infant play brings to everyone's mind is the *freedom* it allows to experiment and express.[6] It is also the first of the traits marked by Caillois, who here is influenced by Huizinga. He stresses that as controlled play is no longer play, it loses its nature of attractive and joyful fun. Interestingly for the purposes of LUDI, Caillois gives to the construct of freedom, more properly, the meaning of spontaneity, immediacy, carefreeness, means of desire and action: "a basic freedom is central to play in order to stimulate distraction and fantasy. This liberty is its indispensable motive power and is basic to the most complex and carefully organized forms of play. Such a primary power of improvisation and joy, which I call *paidia*, is allied to the taste for gratuitous difficulty that I propose to call *ludus*" (Caillois, 2001:27). But to Caillois, play is free also because it can only belong to free men: "it is a luxury activity and it belongs to free men. Hungry people don't play" (ibid:14).

Freedom in play has also overlooked implications, perhaps slightly embarrassing, in field studies; in fact, it also means license and licentiousness: in play gestures and words, and in jokes and diatribes. Sutton-Smith, in this regard, underlines the extreme aspect that these kinds of play may show: "At the very least, they suggest that for the children who take part in the jokery, there need be no limit to the shocks they can include in this kind of unorthodox play—so long as they make them funny" (Sutton-Smith, 2008: 91).

The characteristic of freedom often made it possible to counterpoise play to work, both in the case of the activities of children and adults, and in the case of leisure time and organised time, for example, through pedagogical activities. However, freedom is never associated with laziness or boredom, but rather with *concentration*, *intensity*, and *density*; and these are additional notable features of our object of study. Poetic expressions have been used to describe the condition in which a child plays: if Fink (1960) talks about dense reality, where life is highly concentrated and children appear to be totally absorbed by it, Huizinga talks about tension, that is the desire to achieve, to be successful, and to interrupt that same tension. But these are conditions that are both powerful and knowledgeable: "Play demonstrates that two different attitudes co-exist: to be fully involved in what one is doing and to be aware of the fact that we are within a relative, delimited and conditioned dimension" (Besio, 2008: 1).

According to Huizinga, "this intensity of, and absorption in, play finds no explanation in biological analysis. Yet in this intensity, this absorption, this power of maddening, lies the very essence, the primordial quality of play" (Huizinga, 1938:3). Nature might have given to her children the power of "discharging superabundant

6 Vygotskij (1967) contrasts this interpretation by putting the bond, the limit, at the basis of the pleasure inherent to play.

energy, of relaxing after exertion"; but "no, she gave us play, with its tension, its mirth, and its fun" (ibidem).

Here is another important characteristic of play: it is, in fact, always associated with *fun* and/or *pleasure*. According to Freud (1920), play responds, is led by the "principle of pleasure", which first appears in the children's ludic activities: in his famous example of the nephew who enjoys playing toss and catch with a spool whenever the mother leaves the room, he sees the proof that the child feels joy in anticipating or representing the possible, desired, return of his mother. The active role exercised by the child acting on the spool allows the desire to materialise, and the child to dominate an unpleasant emotion—which is no longer passively suffered—and replacing it with a pleasant one.[7]

The pleasure produced by play does not seem to run out spontaneously in the excitement of the moment, an end in itself; on the contrary, it seems to leave traces, an imprint on the individual's feelings in relation to life itself: "[play's positive pleasure] makes it possible to live more fully in the world, no matter how boring or painful or even dangerous ordinary reality might seem" (Sutton-Smith, 2008:95).

Although sometimes play, in its beautiful swing between opposites, positively makes use of the scheme, the repetition, the use of known and familiar, its underlying backbone lies in what is new, in discontinuity.[8] In fact, it pursues and uses flexibility: not only does it tend towards reproduction, imitation, but it constantly seeks changes, "in form or in content. Play is a phenomenon to the extent of what is possible" (Bondioli, 2002:55).[9]

Fun comes often from the unexpected, from *surprise* (Eberle, 2014): here are some of the attributes of play listed by Sutton-Smith: chanciness, fluidity, ambiguity, particularity, diversity of perspective (Henricks, 2015:117). Teasing, a specific type of play studied by this author, seems to be specifically related to the feeling of surprise or even shock; it takes different forms according to the cultures in which it can be found, and it seems relevant in the play relationship between the child and the adult, becoming a means of social learning.

Even if it happens often, fun does not necessarily, however, become laughter, joy, relief, or cheerfulness, or even sometimes excitement: "Of course, it must be stressed that the pleasure of play is not always manifested in delight or glee or laughter. Play, as Huizinga (1967) points out at great length, can be a very *serious* business but still

7 This wish, according to Freud, is a wish to be adults and to act like them (Metra, 2006).

8 With reference to a sociological perspective, Sutton-Smith adds: "The challenge for scholars is to explain the social, personal and cultural implications of this quest for disorder, excitement, and disconnection. [...] One can also look at all kinds of games [...], as well as at all of the play in the arts [...] and see that in all of them the world is a more exciting place in which to live for a player or spectator, at least for a time" (Sutton-Smith, 2015: 249).

9 All quotations of Italian authors have been translated by the author of this chapter.

within play the act of doing is clearly rewarding in the sense that it incites its own repetition" (Miller, 1973:91).

The play in which the child is involved is always seriously *challenging*,[10] driven by *intrinsic motivation* not only or not so much to achieve a result, but rather to keep alive the play process itself and to continue to belong to it, along with fellow players, if any. According to Miller, both the practice play and rule-based play or team game provide the same pleasure of 'being in' the play, rather than to achieve a result. Winning a game or achieving a result is "important insofar as they are symbols for the dynamics and the challenge that were involved in their attainment" (ibid:93).

Play ends and finds meaning in itself, therefore, in the pleasure of doing and the process of playing;[11] "The interest of the subject is addressed to the process rather than to the product; the usual means-ends relationship is reversed. In other words, the game is intrinsically motivated, does not tend to satisfy primary physical needs, and does not depend on external rules or social obligations. The presence of rules does not contradict the principle of freedom, as submission to the ludic conventions takes place thanks to autonomous choice" (Bondioli, 2002:55).

Play is a challenging process and from the player—child or adult—demands commitment and seriousness (a careless player is reprimanded by his or her companions and is asked to 'play for real'). But, notes Bondioli, the dividing line between play, especially that of fiction, and reality must always be clearly maintained: "The seriousness with which the child or the adult takes their games and their pastimes, the fact that play often requires compliance with detailed rules and procedures, does not eliminate the 'not serious' quality of these activities in relation to ordinary life. The confusion between the two plans is not allowed: the children are reprimanded or reassured if they take their play too seriously; they are reminded that *it is just a game*"(ibid:40). In fiction or in playful concentration, several 'make-believe' acts are accomplished 'seriously', but the realism of such acts must never let the two contexts overlap.

1.3 Fundamentals of Play

A ludic activity has many facets and has been described under many aspects. In this section, an attempt is made to identify and describe some essential parameters of

10 It seems important to point out that Milner (1952), quoted by Winnicott (1971), proposed a connection between children's play and adults' concentration.

11 Some authors speak of 'autotelic activities'. In his well-known *theory of flow*, Csikszentmihalyi (1990; 1997) increasingly uses the term 'autotelic activity' instead of 'playful activities' or play. And, Suits proposes one of the shortest existing definitions of play as follows: "a temporary reallocation to autotelic activities of resources primarily committed to instrumental purposes" (Suits, 1977:124).

the phenomenon, as it manifests in childhood that should be considered crucial for studying play by children with disabilities.

Six fundamental have been identified in the related fields and will be discussed in their various facets, in what follows, with respect to the existing literature, they are: the concept of *frame* and of *being involved*, the need of *doing*, the role of *imagination* and *fantasy*, the importance of the *rules*, the *social aspects* of play, its *capacity to evolve* in childhood.

The first fundamental of play to be considered is the special condition of life that is experienced and acted during this activity: this experience can be defined as *being in the game*, or *in-lusio* (Huizinga, 1967). Play, as inlusio—Latin origin of the word—is "a transformation of reality into a hypothetical connection, without claims to objectivity: it moves away from reality, but it does not transcend it" (Gily, 2006).

Bateson (1956) identified and highlighted this feature of play as a *frame* better and before other authors. "Play is a context, or what Bateson calls a 'frame'. It is a mode of organization of behaviour—one way of fitting pieces of activity together" (Miller, 1973:92).

The essence of play is in its being a meta-communication; a player must be able to state: "This is play". This message creates a frame, a psychological framework, serving as a filter for the interpretation of what there is inside. By playing, one gets into a context and into a dimension different from reality, governed by specific rules, shared by and known to players; play implies a change of perspective, or rather, of paradigm.[12]

By playing, one makes a logical leap, from learning a content (a 'type one' learning) to 'deutero learning', which concerns contexts, relationships, and their modes of functioning. It is in this sense that Bateson can highlight the *paradoxical feature* of play: it requires an agreement among players on what 'is true' and what 'is make believe'; the parties must agree on the framework within which they find themselves, by defining the ludic status of their activity, and maintaining it as it is during its development (Bondioli, 2002).

The players agree willingly and quickly, and show a common desire to inhabit that frame, to indeed 'be in play'; they defend their ludic activity against intruders, who would like to introduce a coherence criterion, unrelated to the proposed rules, because they don't want play to distort into something different. If a child violates the rules and does not seem really involved in play, he or she is considered a troublemaker,[13] and is, in fact, ruled out, or play disappears. But play is not totally an illusion, because it is not confused with the real data, thus generating misunderstandings; to

---

12 Bateson himself refers to the notion of paradigm in Kuhn.

13 Bondioli (2002) refers to a story—entitled *Childhood*—by Tolstoj, in which he vividly describes his brother's listless participation in collective play.

stop it, another meta-communication should happen—"I won't play any more"—that dissolves the frame, the previously established scenario.

A second fundamental aspect that is necessary to highlight concerns the theme of *doing*, and its relationships between means and ends, within the play activity. It was Winnicott who declared the game inseparable from doing. Postulating an indeterminate place between an 'inside' of the child—without further defining it—and an 'outside' where what for him or her is a 'not-me', the author points out that "to control what is outside, one has to *do things*, not simply to think or to wish, and *doing things takes time*. Playing is doing" (1971:41).[14] Winnicott refers here to a third potential space between the mother and the child, which is not the inside or the outside, in which the objects and the transitional phenomena may be acted out and do their job of separation. This area is indeed experiential.[15]

What is interesting to point out here is the emphasis Winnicott places on doing, on action, in a space and a time that are specifically created; this 'doing' has very specific characteristics, which have been well studied by Miller (1973) and concern the relationship between means and ends.

Focussing first on practice play,[16] the author highlights three important aspects, related to his notion of 'galumphing'[17]: a) "a lack of streamlining or task oriented efficiency" (ibid:91), it seems that children deliberately complicate their play activities, they make things difficult for themselves;[18] b) play "is pre-exercise of undeveloped skills that will be needed later. The skills used in practice play are played with after they are acquired. They may not have been completely mastered, but some amount of competence must already have been attained. Practice play can certainly be exercise, but it is more often post-exercise than pre-exercise" (ibid:91); and c) when activities appear in the learning or in the task mode, they are "under the control of goals: means are marshalled at the service of ends. In play, the means are given much freer sway. The process becomes play when it becomes interesting in itself. It is repeated and repeated, and then some part or new consequence of the process becomes the object of interest and is elaborated in its turn. The distinction between process and end state is an important one" (ibid:91).

---

14 This assertion of Winnicott, in particular, has triggered numerous applicative studies of play, in psychotherapy, but also in education, based precisely on the ludic value of 'doing'.

15 It is the "third part of the life of a human being, a part that we cannot ignore, an intermediate area of experiencing, to which inner reality and external both contribute" (Winnicott, 1971:3).

16 With reference to the first developmental stage of play proposed by Piaget (1972).

17 The author admits to use the "appropriately ridiculous term 'galumphing' [...] as an onomatopoetic description of a baboon's flailing in play fights. [...] I will use 'galumphing' as a shorthand term for 'patterned, voluntary elaboration or complication of process, where the pattern is not under the dominant control of goals'" (Miller, 1973:92).

18 This is underlined also by Groos (1901), who speaks about "a process in which the player sets obstacles in his path to prolong and increase the enjoyment of his play" (cited in Miller, 1973:91).

Fun solicited by practice play—one of the main characteristics of play mentioned in the previous paragraph—is a sort of gratification pleasure: “The fun of practice play is most concisely described by Buhler (1930) as Funktionslust—functional pleasure. It is a pleasure of doing, of the act of producing an effect, not of attaining the effect or result itself” (ibid:91).

Afterwards, in his study, the author maintains that the other two Piagetian types of play, that is, rule-based play and symbolic play, cause the same functional pleasure in relation to the process rather than the goals. In fact: “the goal of a game like baseball or chess is by itself meaningless—it attains meaning and motivational value as it is magnified by the lengthening and elaboration of the path that leads to it”. Since, according to him, “the difference between symbolic and rule-bound games is one of form and of the source of the patterns along which the player elaborates his action”, the assumption also applies to symbolic play. The thesis maintained by the author on the reversal of the means/ends relationship in the ludic activity is not only particularly attractive for the underlining feature of autotelic play, but also because from here, Miller draws arguments for the role play can assume as an adaptive function.

But another crucial aspect of the action in play is that children usually impose constraints, obstacles, limitations to their play activities, in order to make them more interesting, more fun. Acting is more desirable if it is imposed by oneself: “But clearly there is somehow something very desirable about acting, at least for a time, in a framework designed by ourselves rather than by the existential forces that run most of our life” (ibid:97).

Ellis views play as a word useful to “categorize behaviours that elevate arousal” (Ellis, 1973:107); but individuals try to assure themselves that they are in control of those arousal-seeking processes. According to White (1959), in fact, creatures try to position themselves within “a protected occasion that contains both familiar and unfamiliar elements and that possesses problems or challenges they consider intriguing or significant. In this light, play activities seem self-motivated attempts to create and solve problems” (Henricks, 2015:2).

This is true at every level and in every type of play, ending up an interesting element of the feeling of challenge that pertains to play, and constituting for some authors, first of all Sutton-Smith (2008), one of the numerous ‘dual’ or better yet ‘dualudic’ elements that form the ‘multiplex functions’ of play.

A fundamental factor of play of huge significance, perhaps the first one that comes immediately to mind when talking about children’s play, is the role of *imagination* and *fantasy*, of the ‘pretend’, or the symbol if you want. In short, we might say, the relationship between the real and the unreal; or, in Erikson’s words, “a step sidewards into another reality”[19] (Erikson, 1963:221-222).

---

19 Actually, this sentence refers to the play of adults; the author, in fact, continues: “The playing adult steps sideward into another reality; the playing child advances forward to new stages of mastery”.

The importance of symbolic in play for Piaget is well known, and so much so as to induce him to devote an entire stage of child's play; he considers it as an inevitable consequence of the fact that play is driven by the process of assimilation,[20] and that among the attributes of the latter, there is distortion: "as soon as we leave the sensorimotor level to the representational thought" (Piaget, 1976:679) the phenomenon of symbolism manifests itself.

Unlike the previous stage—practice play—symbolic play gradually disengages from the frequent link with repetition, and some daily behaviours appear unrelated to their original purpose, simply by evocation. Repetition without a purpose is used to disengage the representation from the evocative situation, and then to be free to combine the representations in a form that anticipates thought.

The schemes drawn from real life are first applied to inadequate objects and later evoked, up to the consciousness of 'pretend'; symbolic play "marks the primacy of the representation both on the action and on the perception as well as of the meaning on the object" (Bondioli, 2002:411). There cannot be pretence before the birth of the representation; it is from pretend play that the real symbol, the language, as well as human creativity, a free combination of symbols, metaphorical transformation of reality, will arise.

However, there is an undeniable relationship, for Piaget, between practice play and symbolic play: "symbolic play is to practice play how the representative intelligence is to sensorimotor intelligence. This matching at two different levels should be added to another at the same level: symbolic play is to representative intelligence how practice play is to sensorimotor intelligence" (Piaget, 1976:690).

Vygotskij (1967; 2004) does not like the expression 'symbolic play' because it is too tied to the semiotic meaning of 'sign', which tends to intellectualise the construct and overly emphasises the cognitive aspects of play, while neglecting the circumstances and motivation. He rather prefers to use the concept of imagination: in establishing some criteria for distinguishing the play of a child from other forms of activity, he concludes that, in play, the child creates an imaginary situation; this is not considered a type of play, but the peculiar characteristic of play in general.

Play is a 'transitional stage' in the development of imagination; in this way, Vygotskij totally reverses a common previous belief that imagination precedes play: "Imagination is a new formation that is not present in the consciousness of the very young child, is totally absent in animals, and represents a specific human form of

20 Assimilation and accommodation are, for Piaget, the two processes that govern the child's adaptation to the environment. Assimilation is the incorporation of an event or an object in a behavioural or cognitive pattern already acquired (for example, the child uses the tail of a puppet like a pillow to lean his or her head on and pretend to sleep). Accommodation guides the modification of the cognitive structure or of the behavioural pattern to include new objects or events yet unknown (e.g., to change a gripping method, to change an approach to a problem). Assimilation and accommodation take turns in search of the necessary homeostasis in the relationship with the environment.

conscious activity. Like all functions of consciousness, it originally arises from action. The old adage that children's play is imagination in action can be reversed: we can say that imagination in adolescents and schoolchildren is play without action" (Vygotskij, 1967:8).

Play is not driven by the symbol, but by desires; the child realises them, puts them into practice, and in this way, the basic categories of reality pass through his or her experience. While thinking, desiring, the child acts. Internal and external action are inseparable: imagination, interpretation, and will are the internal processes brought about by external action; soon the child will not need an object to play, the meaning of the action will become dominant over the real action. This is the way to develop abstract thinking, but also of the will and the ability to choose.

Some objects, however, at least according to Winnicott (1971), are not like the others because they play a special role in the child's development: these objects are symbols, in the sense that they are for something else, namely they 'stand for' the child's mother. They are called transitional objects, and during early childhood, are treated by the child in a special way: they cannot be changed or removed, must be concrete, have a separate existence for the child, but at the same time, they are part of that child. With these objects, the child establishes a relationship, consisting actions that, on the one hand, lets him or her enter the play world, and on the other, allows him or her to experience separation and distance from his or her mother, by representing her through this symbol. It is an object of 'transition', in fact, between self and non-self, between the real and the imagined, just like in make-believe play, where objects are something different and are animated. For Winnicott "the symbolic act is a creative one, that defines a particular dimension of the experience, somewhere between purely subjective reality and objective reality" (Bondioli, 2002:72). The symbolic makes it possible to separate these two worlds and to create a third one, called by Winnicott 'play space' and 'illusion space' (once again in-lusio), a space of the experience that is not given, but is created by the child, as a product of his or her mental activity and of his or her action on reality.

Rules are the fourth fundamental factor of play to be considered: how they arise, their detection, and their role in the child's play development.

One of the basic lines of demarcation in the interpretation of play between the two giants of the field, Piaget and Vygotskij, for example, is placed precisely on this point. For Piaget, according to his theory of child development, pretend play or symbolic play is not based on rules, because the rule is grafted on social skills—for example of bargaining and mediation—which occur only when the phase of egocentrism has been surpassed. Consistently, the author singles out 'rule-based play' as a standalone play stage, the last one in the hierarchy he proposes.

One rule, for Piaget, can exist on an individual basis—thus, it can be changed at will—and has an objectual content (e.g., making a certain number of steps before throwing a ball), or it can have a social basis and result from an agreement between the players, who find a compromise between different wills and intentions—and therefore, it has a binding value. Both types of rules are based on conventionality; thus, they are not compatible with pretend play, which cannot be guided by rules, as it has a subjective nature.

However, Piaget seems to remain isolated with respect to other scholars: in fact, according to Huizinga, for example, every type of play, even pretend play, is characterised by rules: "Rule creates the typical magic circle of play, it allows you to separate the ludic actions from the not-ludic ones, thus creating the inlusio, the feeling of "being in play" (Bondioli, 2002). And Caillois, who keeps the Piagetian meaning of a rule as a convention, however, considers that, in make-believe play, the meaning of 'as if' is to replace the rule and to fulfil the same function.

Vygotskij's position is completely antithetical to Piaget's: the rule is intrinsic to both rule-based play and pretend play;[21] it has an important psycho-developmental function, but also a critical and direct influence on the effectiveness and success of the ludic activity. In fact, it obliges the child not to follow his or her immediate impulses, even by acting against them: within competition games, one must submit to data constraints, in pretend play "the action is subject to the meaning, while, in real life, the action wins out over meaning" (Vygotskij, 1976:552). Thus, Vygotskij can state that, in play, freedom is only illusory: "While playing, children are free, they determine their actions starting from their self. But [...] their actions are subject to a well-defined meaning, and they act according to the meanings of things" (ibidem). For example, the child does not eat a piece of candy if within the play activity it is considered poisoned.

However, self-control of the immediate impulses has a direct consequence on the play activity: "It is in fact through the line of maximum resistance—self-submitting to the rule of giving up spontaneous and impulsive actions—that the maximum of pleasure is achieved in play" (Bondioli, 2002:31). For Vygotskij, "the essential attribute in play is a rule that has become a desire. Spinoza's notion of 'an idea that has become a desire, a concept that has turned into a passion' has its prototype in play, which is the realm of spontaneity and freedom" (Garvey, 1976:580). Play gives the child a new form of desires, it shows him or her how to relate his or her desires with a dummy 'I', with its role in the play activity and with the play rules.

Obviously, the theme of the rule recalls the classical division between play and game. For Geertz (1973) and Caillois, play could result in the game being predominantly made up of rules: "Tout jeux est système de règles... ces conventions sont à la fois arbitraires, impératives et sans appel. Elles ne peuvent être violées sous aucun prétexte, sous peine que le jeu prenne fin sur-le-champ et se trouve détruit par le fait même" (Caillois, 1967; préface). Bateson and Winnicott, however, were primarily interested in the playful dimension of play: "Let's look at what is good and what is bad about 'playing' and 'games'. First of all, I don't mind—not much—about winning

21 Instead, the sensorimotor play of the child's first 3 years remains, according to Vygotskij, without rules.

or losing" (Bateson, 1972:14). Bateson does not play to win, but to create; rules exist because they can be broken and put us in trouble: this is the gist of play, trying to get out of it and finding out which rules are obeyed while playing.

Avedon and Sutton-Smith (1971) described play as a behaviour characterised by the interest in the actions *in se*, *per se*, in which the goal is secondary, individual and not durable; games, on the contrary, have rules and specific purposes and are characterised by repeatable patterns and predictable results. Between game and play, there isn't a relationship during human development because at any age, the child can be involved in play or in games.

Bettelheim (1972; 1984) instead makes a separation; first comes play with self-imposed rules, which does not produce intentional results in the external reality, then the games, which are characterised by agreed-upon rules, often imposed externally, by the need to use tools for their intended use and not by imagination. If the examples of play and games made by Bettelheim make reference to the distinction between pretend play and rule-based play, their respective characteristics are similar to those of Avedon and Sutton-Smith. Also, the transition from play to game seems to be inspired, according to Vygotskij, by an increase in impulse control, by the acquisition of the sense of reality, and social adaptation. Finally, for Bettelheim, games are social materials with an institutional existence; they are a part of tradition and culture.

The fifth characteristic of play concerns the *social aspects* of play, that were already mentioned here, and in particular, were introduced by the Batesonian construct of 'frame'. This theme opens at least two lines of study: on the one hand, the fact that children learn to play, in dual relationships or in group: with siblings, peers, but also with parents and adults.[22] On the other, because most of the types and modes of play create and require social contexts.

Starting from this last aspect, Coplan et al. suggest that play involving dyads or groups can be defined 'social' when the child "(a) is motivated to engage others in playful activities; (b) is able to regulate emotional arousal; (c) possesses the skills necessarily to initiate interactions with another child, such that; (d) the social overtures are accepted in kind" (Coplan et al., 2015:96). Any possible type of play can take place with a social mode; "it also comprises active conversations between children as they go about interacting with each other, negotiating play roles and game rules". On the contrary, "non-social play is defined as the display of solitary activities and behaviours in the presence of other potential play partners". Taxonomies of social play exist; the best known and used in the field have been developed by Parten (1932).[23]

---

22 Including education in formal, non-formal, and informal contexts, for example, the available means of communication.

23 It is based on the following four categories: (1) unoccupied behaviour; (2) onlooker behaviour; (3) solitary play; (4) parallel play.

The importance of the involvement of peers has always been valued in the sector studies; Piaget, for example, "suggested exposure to instances of interpersonal differences of opinion and thought with one's peers (as opposed to interactions with adults) and opportunities for discussion and negotiation about these differences, aided children in the acquisition and development of sensitive perspective-taking skills in interpersonal relationships" (Coplan et al., 2015:99).

This somehow echoes Garvey's definition, which states the social game as "a condition of commitment, in which the successive and abstract behaviours of a partner are contingent to the abstract behaviours of the other. [...] This means leaving space in one's behaviour to the reactions of the other and changing one's own behaviours as a result of the actions of the other" (Garvey, 1976:697).[24]

Peer interaction through play has been considered crucial also for the development of the self-system: "exchanges among peers, in the contexts of cooperation, competition, conflict, and friendly discussion, allowed the child to gain an understanding of the self as both subject and object (the notion of 'looking glass self')" (Coplan et al., 2015:99).[25]

Sullivan (1953) proposed that experiences within the peer group are essential for the development of skills of cooperation, compromise, empathy, and altruism and for the acquisition and maintenance of important social skills of the adult's life. Recent research perspectives focus on the development of children who rarely engage others in social play (Göncü & Gaskins, 2011).

There are marked differences among children in their willingness to engage in social play and in the degree to which they are motivated to take part in peer play. Individual differences are influenced by increasing age, but also by "dispositional characteristics (e.g., temperament, sex), social motivations, social competence" (Coplan et al., 2015:100) and by culture and parental influence.

The influence of a good, supportive, and loving family environment is vital for play to appear in a child's life: Spitz's studies on orphanages (1945) showed that contexts lacking meaningful relationships, care, and emotional support caused serious deprivations in children, even in play. Caring parents know immediately that their child feels pleasure in being stimulated, so they propose the game of 'Cuckoo'; they throw him or her in the air; they surprise him or her with unexpected playful gestures; later they inspire him or her to play, so that he or she can learn; they offer him or her suitable objects, new, different in shape and colour (Petrie, 1987); they also

24 According to him, four possible conditions can be drawn when only two children are together: the non-social game (both can work together to mend a broken toy); the non-game non-social (one or both of them may independently examine an object); playing non-social (one or both can engage in imaginative activity independently); the social game (both are mutually engaged in a shared activity).

25 The reference here is to C. H. Cooley's notion of 'looking glass self' as reported in Mead, G. H. (1934). *Mind, Self and Society*. Chicago: University of Chicago Press.

present them as animating characters; thus, providing an opportunity for starting the pretend play.

Many studies (Schaffer, 1977) led to the belief that children learn to play, especially "by playing with an adult who shows to share the play and the inherent pleasure" (Bondioli, 2002:105). Adults, mothers in the first place, convey to the child the idea that actions can be carried out in many ways, including the pretend one, that objects can represent something else, and that it is possible to do something just to take pleasure in doing it together.

The child's first play activities, ritualised and repetitive, are common in many cultures (playing to hide parts of one's face or objects, performing a series of rhythmic actions on the child's body up to a fast closing and full of excitement, capturing the child's interest and increasing his or her attention time, and so on).

If, at first, the adult is the protagonist and the child the spectator, the roles are reversed quite quickly;[26] this process takes place, thanks to the gradual withdrawal of the adults from their preeminent role, while in the meantime, the child becomes able to promote the ludic activity. Then finally, the adult acts as a mediator of a ludic contact with other children, suggesting and facilitating connections among peers in play.

One of the areas in which the role of the adult as a prompter in play that has been studied in the literature, is role-playing,[27] which is founded and managed on the transmission of scripts; according to Garvey (1982), the required skills in social role-playing are suggested following a modelling procedure that takes place in the home environment: children "in this way should have the occasion to learn: conventional sounds associated with certain gestures of 'pretend play', personification and animation of dolls, specific communication techniques to indicate the make-believe, a processing in a non-literal perspective of roles, scripts and ludic plots" (Bondioli, 2002:111). Also, in this case, the adult gradually disengages from play, becoming just a spectator and intervening if anything to provide new scripts and to introduce more complex ideas (e.g., a state of health of the doll, an unexpected event).

Haight carried out an interesting study on the direct and indirect influence of adults on child's play, and pretend play in particular. Her literature analysis on this theme makes it possible to assert that "parent-child pretend play is a potentially rich context for the socialization and acquisition of cultural meaning" (Haight, 1998:262); parents follow different ways to support their children's play: they can teach them

---

26 Sutton-Smith (1979) indicated the following: 1) routine of exchange, the adult imitates the child and vice versa; 2) the central person's routine: the adult acts, the child serves as co-actor and routine in unison, the actions happen together; 3) the child does something on adult who pretends to withdraw offended, surprised, or scared.

27 Role-playing is an expression that can correspond to different meanings and techniques. In the case of children's play, make-believe can be considered a kind of role playing, whereas they adopt a role—a teacher, a doctor, and so on—and act out as characters in this role.

how to pretend, introduce the pretend mode, elaborate "upon their toddlers early forays into the non-literal"; they also used to encourage children to be enthusiastic about pretend play. However, she also found significant cultural differences, so she concludes: "before advocating parent-child play, practitioners must consider the cultural appropriateness of adult-child play, adults' own preferences for interaction with children, as well as other play and nonplay contexts that may promote similar developmental outcomes" (ibidem).

The research of O'Connell and Bretherton (1984) indicates that children's play is less repetitive, more advanced, and less fragmented initially when they play with an adult rather than with a peer; furthermore, in this case, play can be enriched as to its variety, level, and duration.

In particular, it is interesting to note that though mothers cannot tailor their proposals to the child's potential, they naturally offer a range of possibilities from which the child draws freely, according to his or her wishes and possibilities.

Indispensible elements to support the child's play seems to be emotional support, encouragement, effective participation in recreational settings; furthermore, the interaction style must maintain a delicate balance between stimulation and non-interference.

The last, but really not the least, characteristic of play considered here concerns the fact that its *capacity to evolve* in childhood; the child's play modalities, the proposals he or she advances or to whom he or she is able to answer, the areas of interest he or she develops, and in correlation, the ludic activities he or she does, change over time, from birth to 18 years.[28] The study of this evolution has involved all scholars in the field, who have proposed different classifications, identifying types and categories of play in correlation with the respective epistemological frameworks of reference.

A careful and detailed examination of proposed classifications of play is presented in this text, Chapter 3, which should be consulted for a more in-depth analysis.

Therefore, the development of play is still considered a useful indicator of a child's development, and to such a degree that it is also used as a diagnostic tool in some cases to identify growth-related problems.

What is worth noting here is the contrast between two main approaches: on the one hand, that of the successive stages of play—of which the Piagetian one is certainly the best known—which proposes a hierarchical alternation between the stages of play; each stage develops and grows in complexity, then exhausts its developmental function for the individual and is replaced by the following one, which in turn

---

28 The theme of the relationship between the concepts of play and the concepts of time was discussed in an original way by Henricks (2009). According to this approach, we are undoubtedly referring here to the concept of 'play as progress'. A detailed examination of studies about the evolution of play is presented in Chapter 3.

maintains with the previous one more or less direct and recognisable relationship; and on the other hand, there is the approach inspired by cultural psychology and then by constructivism, that while identifying an evolution—not rigidly hierarchical—in characteristics, types, and degrees of complexity of children's play, enhances the value of inter-individual variability, avoids the correlation between type of play, and predefined chronological ages of the child and does not support the idea of a linear progression between stages (Rubin et al., 1983). Moreover, it points out the influence of many concomitant factors, and not only of the cognitive ones: desires, volitions, emotions, experiences, and social contexts of life.[29]

In the first case, play is connected to an epistemology which provides "invariant and qualitative different stages of development; such stages are typically cumulative, in that later ones build off earlier levels. Furthermore, later stages are thought to be more complex, rationally controlled and abstract. Indeed, human development itself is sometimes equated to the creation and maintenance of personal schemas that feature increasing degrees of integration and control" (Henricks, 2009:16).

Play develops and proceeds from stage to stage, according to Piaget, substantially thanks to intellectual development, with which it is considered closely related, since its inception.

The practice play of infancy becomes "more sophisticated as the child's ability to act intelligently develops. When children's sensory-motor schemes become sufficiently coordinated to construct the concept of object permanence, the ability to represent absent realities becomes possible" (De Lisi, 2015:235). During growth, "intellectual development from early to late childhood includes an increasing ability to mentally coordinate concepts that are needed to adapt to the natural, physical and social worlds. These changes have an effect on children's symbolic play. As children come to understand the importance of reciprocity in relationships (especially as experienced in peer relationships), they develop a deeper understanding of the necessity to conform to social rules and conventions, including following the rules in games" (ibidem).

The second case can be found typically in Vygotskij's original interpretation. His core idea is that "the history of human development is a complex interplay between the processes of natural development that are determined biologically and the processes of cultural development brought about by the interaction of the growing individual with other people" (Bodrova & Leong, 2015:204).

Vygotskij explains exactly this way the birth and development of high mental functions, in his view poorly studied by earlier theories: they appear and are built first within social relations in which the child is immersed, and secondly, they become psychological and biological functions of the individual. To put it directly in

29 An interesting analysis of the concept of 'stage' in the constructivist epistemology can be found in Marshall (2009).

his own words: “Every function in the cultural development of the child appears on the stage twice, in two planes, first, the social, then the psychological, first between people as an ‘inter’ mental category, then within the child as ‘intra’ mental category. This pertains equally to voluntary attention, to logical memory, to the formation of concepts and to the development of will” (Vygotskij, 1997:136).

It is exactly the role played by the social context and relationships that belong to it that allows Vygotskij to lay the foundations for one of the most famous and compelling concepts of his entire theoretical framework: “the Zone of Proximal Development (ZPD) [which is] the distance between the level of independent performance and the level of assisted performance” (Bodrova & Leong, 2015:206). Vygotskij’s idea is that play creates the ZPD of a child, and that play is the leading activity for children of preschool and kindergarten age.[30] Within the ZPD, the entire child’s development takes place, and in this sense, it is possible to state that it is play that creates development.

The study of the evolutionary nature of play and the analysis of its effective evolution in subsequent stages have always attracted scholars in the field. The three typologies proposed by Piaget have formed an essential basis for everyone, to break it away and articulate it, making it more comprehensive and complex. The classifications of the types of play, whether or not included in the frameworks of child development, are now numerous, and are treated in more detail in Chapter 3.

The flourishing of these proposals appears to be due to a latent dissatisfaction with the completeness of the existing classifications; thanks to the careful observation of children’s play lasting decades, radical ruptures between one stage (or type) and another cannot be acceptable, because they seem rather to merge, each feeding the other, to resurrect in different forms, in different times of life; and yet educators, psychologists, and experts in general in the play field feel the need to have, know, and distinguish them.

Some examples may be useful to highlight these aspects.

The baby’s body is certainly one of the first objects with which he or she plays (Garner & Bergen, 2015), during the stage of practice play: his or her own feet, his or her own hands assume for him or her a special interest, because they can act, set in motion, and provoke interesting feelings; this play becomes more complex in the following months, as the body comes in contact with the world that must be explored, crossed. But later, much later, the body itself will become a symbol, when it will be used to imitate the actions of the adults at a distance, or even later when it is masked or brought on a stage, moving towards a more frankly symbolic phase.

---

30 “This laid the foundation of the theories of play developed by the so-called post-Vygotskian scholars. [...] all these theories put emphasis on play not as a reflection of past experiences but rather as the activity essential for the development of a ‘future child’” (Bodrova & Leong, 2015:207).

The constructive game, from Smilansky on (1968), has acquired—despite some controversy—the dignity of a special type of play, creeping in between practice play and symbolic play: it requires complex psychomotor skills—both for precisely managing small elements to be assembled as in the case of Lego bricks, and for giving life to toys and real worlds, for example, a rudimentary canoe, a platform on a tree—which cannot be included within the group of the approximate abilities of practice play; and it also, very often, requires an ability to hypothesise work plans, monitor their implementation, if necessary, undo and redo again. In the case of creating worlds with their own characters and stories, constructive play intertwines with symbolic play and adopts the peculiarities of this play type, becoming, perhaps, something else.

Another possible example is exercise, exploratory and gym play with the abilities of the body that the child demonstrates on the playground: this can only be classified as practice play, because new psychomotor skills are continuously refined during actions and in relationship with objects of different shapes and nature; yet, it engages children of all ages, sometimes it even becomes an enticement for adults. When it assumes the form of a race or a competition, it also makes use of rules that can be agreed upon or the result of mediation.

Moreover, most of the video games, and some so-called 'educational games' for early childhood, are merely practice play applied to a task: to perfectly carry out coordinated fine, sometimes minimal movements; from the cognitive point of view, they propose the endless repetition of the solution to the same problem.[31] In some cases, these over-specialised psychomotor skills can be used to play video games with rules and strategies.

Caillois' proposal (1958) can be considered, at least partially, consonant with the need not to consider the types of play as rigidly determined; certainly it stands out among other proposals for its originality and impressive reach. His well-known taxonomy does not concern the types of play, but rather the player's disposition. The four identified dimensions are not mutually exclusive, but rather can be present together and aspire to exhaust all possible types of play: *agon*, or competition (the play done by two or more participants, where there is someone who wins and someone who loses: running, playing ball, wrestling, billiards, chess); *alea*, or chance (again, play involving a number of persons, but based on the role of chance: to see who is going to be 'it', bingo, lottery, gambling); *mimos*, or imitation, simulacrum (pretending, masks, theatre); *ilinx*, or vertigo, vortex (the swing, dancing, mountain climbing). These four dimensions are moving, however,

31 This is the case of toys like 'Sapientino', which awards the association between the same pairs—for example, of images—but also of many electronic games and the so-called educational software based merely on the relationship between cause and effect (push a button, turn a lever, select an area of the monitor to achieve a given and known scope).

along two fundamental and different levels of tension, to 'being in the play': they are *paidia*—a 'first, primary freedom', the unrestrained imagination typical of younger children, but existing in varying degrees in any recreational activity—and *ludus*—rule-based play, more related to adulthood; however, the two levels are placed at opposite ends of a continuum, and all play activities will include different grades of these dimensions, mixing them.

The proposal of Caillois offers a series of elements that can be combined in various sizes and degrees of intensity of the personal involvement. But it does not take into account directly and specifically the issue of play development, of the changes it undergoes during the individual's life.

The identification of different types of play, their emergence in different periods of the individual's development, together with their growing complexities and intertwining over time are matters of specific interest for those wishing to explore play as a specific topic of interest in the field of education—and in case of children with disabilities, also of rehabilitation. A deeper awareness on the play development, in fact, gives the educators and the adults in general the opportunity to knowingly extend the proposals of play activities, as to the settings, the mediators, the relationships, and of course, the type and the complexity.

Summarising here the strengths of the existing proposals and the analysed criticisms, one might conclude that a model of interpretation and classification organised in stages, while having the advantage of identifying types, with perspicuity, that are now consolidated in the literature, also introduces a rigidity in the analysis of the phenomenon—for example, the clearly defined stages associated with a specific chronological age, stable and unique over time—for which it is not possible to really understand it and to use it effectively.

It seems more effective and productive to adopt a model that, based on the four main types today—in principle—shared in the field,[32] makes it possible to respect and safeguard the following data: a) in case of regular conditions of development, and environmental or socio-cultural contexts, each type has a peculiar onset in a precise developmental age; b) there is a characteristic progression between the types of play, during development; c) environmental contexts or other technological innovations may give rise to new types of play, which are an amalgam between those already known, with varying degrees of involvement of their characteristics, or different degrees of use of the related skills; d) the types of play can coexist in different stages of life; e) each type of play can be reactivated, reveal itself anew, in different developmental stages, remodelled and recontextualised or simply reproduced by pure ludic spirit.

Play requires, claims, and builds up different competences and abilities during development; it manifests immediately, co-evolves with the child, benefits from new

32 The framework adopted by LUDI is presented in Chapter 3.

skills becoming more and more complex, offering increasingly greater challenges, and stimulating the construction of new—cognitive and social—skills.

It is for this reason that the play classifications 'in separate stages' do not work. They never prove there is a real separation of competences and activities between stages because a new play stage involves the competences of the previous one without exhausting them: on the contrary, it re-elaborates and readjusts them at a new level. At that point, those competences are no longer the same; they are contaminated, more complex, and new.[33]

A graphical representation of this proposed model would probably not be a continuum of a unidirectional timeline, but rather a spiral line, showing the different periods of onset, the progression of the types, their possible coexistence in time, but also the possible contaminations between them and even the somewhat reworked reactivations of some of them, in other periods.

1.4 Functions of Play

But why do people play? To which needs does this activity respond? Which adaptive functions does it support, being so deeply rooted—in time and in space—stable but also changing, transmitted, known?

Scholars have always wondered about the meaning and purpose of this activity, and have advanced explanations on its ultimate meaning, particularly on its role in child's development, where it seems to take precedence and have special meaning. The ludic activity has been mainly studied not "'as such', but as a 'symptom' or a sign of the peculiarity of the infant psyche or mind; play is a paradigmatic phenomenon that sheds light into the world of childhood" (Bondioli, 2009:19).

From time to time, according to an essentially reductionist approach,[34] various functions of play have been highlighted (and will be shortly presented in this paragraph): the biological-adaptive, the cognitive, and the socio-relational, the psycho-emotional.

Some functions of play will now be described and analysed: understanding the possible reasons of play, perceiving the functions it performs in human development,

33 A reference to the representational redescription proposed by Karmiloff Smith (1992) can be found in this description of the evolution of play, as in other expressions of human development, it is possible here to recognise the role played by this process: an alternation between the acquisition of competences, their representative metabolisation and their re-use with a new awareness and new effectiveness.

34 According to Bondioli, the assumption of play within the theories of development meets the criticism of reductionism; in fact, some aspects of the phenomenon are emphasised and used so as to show or prove, following an analogical procedure, some aspects of the epistemological and interpretative models that the different authors would adopt (Bondioli, 2009:19).

can provide support and nourishment to the educational field, including the area of disability.

Almost all researchers mention that the ludic activity does not belong only to human beings, and that some classes of animals[35] devote part of their time, especially puppies, to play in pairs or in groups, with adults and peers. Often these kinds of play involve the carrying out—but in a less precise, less powerful, and less realistic manner—of the animals' daily life movements and actions: fighting, taking care of their puppies, and so on.

These considerations suggested to many authors the idea that play should have a *useful role in ontogenesis*, and also *in phylogeny*; for Kant, it would serve to train the child in activities that ensure preservation of the organism; for Claparède, it is a sort of preparatory exercise; for Groos, an activity able to test skills useful for environmental adaptation; for Fröbel, the expression of the innate creative attitude of human beings—thus almost already a job—and for Carr, a complementary exercise to maintain useful habits that otherwise would disappear.

According to Lorenz, play has an *adaptive function* to explore new situations in new environments, looking for optimal solutions. Miller, in a more systematic way, comes to a similar conclusion: starting from the study of baboons, he claims that play serves to provide a flexible substrate to the individual's cognitive system: "a general ability to produce the novel, an ability that is surely as important to survival as the ability to produce the expected". When people spend their time immersed in a game, "they are creating novelty, however unimposing it might be [...]. It is the habit of occasionally creating novelty, rather than specific preparation, that makes us seem intelligent when, confronted with a new problem, a new contingency in 'reality', we have more than a random chance of marshalling the means at our disposal in a hitherto useless but now adaptive way" (Miller, 1973:96). It cannot be overlooked that Sutton-Smith (1997) argues that "as a form of mental feedback, play might nullify the rigidity that sets in after successful adaption, thus reinforcing animal and human variability".

Also, Huizinga (1938) starts his discourse from the animal experience, noting, however, that play goes beyond the limits of biological experience, as it is a function that contains a meaning; it characterises the *homo ludens*, as a cultural animal: culture itself rises in a playful shape, culture is first played. Play would have the original function of being *a creator of culture*; it opens up the possibility, exquisitely human,

35 Today, ethologists claim that only in the classes of mammals and birds, it is possible to find play as such. Social play is the most common among animals (grapple fights, chases, forms of sexual behaviours, rearing offspring, and so on). Individual play consists exploration and manipulation of objects, motor acrobatics, and pursuits of preys (real and fictional). Apes, if raised in contact with human beings, play in an unusual manner, such as making funny faces in front of a mirror, walking while covering their eyes with a hand to make it more difficult to walk on suspended logs, and doing complex play activities with objects.

to attribute meanings, to comment, making it possible to develop art, science, history, humour. “Not so much rules, behaviour and social roles would be learned through play, but rather the fact that any behaviour has its own context, that it is culturally determined” (Bondioli, 2002:56).

This cultural context, seen, however, exactly as a frame of roles and behaviours, is the interpretation proposed by Bateson: what the child learns from play is not how to behave according to certain rules or roles, but rather that there are types of roles and categories of rules. The child acquires knowledge about the possible roles and styles of behaviour and acquires flexibility regarding the ability to choose and adopt different styles in relation to different frameworks or contexts of behaviour.

The function of play to *support sensorimotor development* has been emphasised since the earliest field studies: the exploration and use of objects—including one’s own body—typical of the *practice play* stage, allow the child to refine sensorimotor coordination and its control, through feedback, hence stabilising processes that gradually become automatic; manipulation and construction of objects become gradually more and more linked to the achievement of objectives and to the action on the surrounding world, thus promoting the use of mental patterns of planning, while manual coordination becomes refined and precise, quickly opening the road to constructive play. Exploration and action on objects create a new mobility of knowledge patterns, which is of great importance for psychological growth.

In these activities, the child always tends to reach greater skills in using objects that attract his or her attention and interest, and for this purpose, he or she constantly alternates tireless repetition of the same gestures and voluntary introduction of constraints, obstacles, and new ways to do things, thus checking the possible changes in the gestures themselves.

Play has also been seen as an engine for *cognitive development*, in all its facets. *Symbolic play* carries out, in this regard, an important function, because it is the evidence of the birth of thought, which detaches from the concrete and the real to start imagination and fancy; it forms the substrate for the development of higher symbolic functions: language, graphical representation, narrative ability.

An interesting aspect of symbolic play—highlighted by Vygotskij—is the fact that it is already sensitive to the effects of rules: players adhere to the constraints of the ‘pretend’, enter in a scheme that is ‘other’ than reality: and this requires the control of two different contexts—reality and pretending—with their respective differences in roles and behavioural patterns; “pretending or not pretending is an experiential duality; [...] these pretend ludic worlds will educate the players in the semantics of the subjective-objective duality destined to occupy their minds forever afterwards” (Sutton-Smith, 2008:119).

Important consequences derive from the symbolic transformation of the real; in particular, the nature and function of play conventions can be learned or reinvented: rule-based play becomes gradually, among the other types of play, the more complex and abstract one, with regard to the cognitive domain; play turns into games, until it is possible to manage entire systems of rules, including strategy and planning games. Moreover, according to Bruner (1986), while teaching, conventions play can teach skills useful for growth and becoming an adult.

However, symbolic play and rule-based play also highlight another fundamental aspect of play, the *development of social skills*. More than the others, these types of play, in fact, open up to social relationships, dual or in group, thus to the ability to share, mediate, recognise, and adhere to social conventions; at this stage, social adaptation is also accompanied by a greater ability to control impulses and a sense of reality.

But play is certainly not just reasoning, social life, real life. Play also belongs, and not for a small part, to the individual's intrapsychic world; indeed, most of the scholars at the beginning of the last century focused on this influence of play on the child's *psychological and emotional development*, and has rekindled the interest of researchers in recent years.[36]

While many authors have seen in play the natural outburst of an overload of emotions carried by the child, for Vygotskij, on the contrary, it gives the child exactly an opportunity to act and experiment the ability to control emotions; imagination itself arises when it is time to ask the child to delay the achievement of immediate pleasure. Again, rules and constraints become extraordinarily important in this case: the pleasure associated with play, in fact, is exactly due to the restrictions voluntarily imposed on the ludic activity. "Play would represent the ideal of Spinoza's 'inner rule', or, to quote Piaget, a rule of self-restraint and self-determination" (Bondioli, 2002:36).

Far removed from these interpretations of the function of play, in relation to the individual's intrapsychic development, comes from the psychoanalytic line of research. Fear, anger, desire, love, ambition, conflict, rivalry are, according to the psychoanalytic theory, the dynamic elements of play, without which it would have no reason to exist. The symbolic act is a substitution act; when the young child sucks his or her thumb even if not hungry, he or she shows one of the primitive phenomena of transient symbolisation, which creates a bridge between the child and the mother when their separation starts. The transitional object—a blanket, a small toy, an object of real life—according to Winnicott's well-known analysis, 'stands for' the mother without being her: it is the first symbol in the child's life, who perceives it at the same time as part of him or her or self, and as separate from him or her or self, independent; by acting on and with the object the separation process starts and proceeds.

36 Fein, for example, offers a synthesis between approaches to play oriented towards cognitive development and emotional development; in her opinion, around 3 years of age, a representative system in two layers has begun developing, one for practical knowledge and the other for affective knowledge, which "makes it possible for the individual to become aware of his/her own inner life and to acquire control on the way to express it" (Fein, 1987:287).

Many other scholars faced this issue, which could be called the relationship between 'identification' and 'separation'; for them, play is not interesting as a form, or as a function, rather its contents should be the subject of interest and study, because they consist of feelings and emotions: "play is a theatre, an enactment, in which an attempt to integrate the emotional experience, thus the self and the world, is implemented. [...] It is a way to cope, to control, to give meaning to the process of growth, seen as dramatically uneven and painful" (Bondioli, 2002:77). These feelings and emotions help the child to adapt to reality and deal with the problems that he or she encounters in real life: "This is an experience that allows the child to check his/her phantasmal events and vicissitudes, on a manipulated and controlled reality, in an illusory dimension (and real together), which favours both an examination of reality and the exercise of concrete skills with a focus on adaptation" (Fornari, 1988:138).

Winnicott describes this path, which develops through the exploration, the knowledge and the use of objects, but above all, through transactional objects, as a passage from "a state of total fusion with the mother to one in which the child begins to be aware of his/her individuality; [...] from a state of primary integration, in which everything that will became later an 'I' is a set of fragmented and disconnected sensations, to a state of integration, characterized by the perception of having an 'inside' and an 'outside'; [...] from a state of absolute dependence (viewed nonetheless as omnipotence) to a state of independence (which involves awareness of limits and dependence). It is a journey which, while leading to the construction and the discovery of the self, also enables the discovery and the construction of the Other from many points of view: social (the one/s with whom it is possible to relate), intellectual (the object of knowledge), affective (the source of pleasure or displeasure)" (Bondioli, 2002:67).

It was Sutton-Smith to push this interpretation—in his usual 'irreverent' style—up to reflecting on the consequences that the ludic activity may have in building the individual's feeling of independence; by playing, perhaps, the children "are protecting themselves against varying hegemonic physical and human realities by making fun of them with these relatively obnoxious representations. There is a kind of courageous parody here", to come to watch play "as at heart a kind of transcendence" (Sutton-Smith, 2008:96).

1.5 Play and Education: the Need for Play for the Sake of Play

Play is a pedagogical topos and an explanation of childhood. The time a child devotes to it, the intensity of his or her concentration while playing, the absoluteness of the emotions that this activity visibly stimulates, the flexibility it demonstrates in changing according to the variation in ages, environmental conditions, companions and constraints, the stability with which it occurs in every geographical area, in every era and every culture, all these features have given play a special status in this unique period of human life called *childhood*.

1.5.1 A Short Historical Overview[37]

Children and adults of all periods have played and have made toys. Egyptians made dolls from cloth or majolica, as well as wooden or stone toys, while Romans made sweets in the form of letters and invented games involving imitation and comparison. Play was used by the Greeks and Romans as a prize following educational activities, and the close link between school and play is also etymologically demonstrated by the two words *skholé* ('fun', 'leisure time' but also 'school' for the Greeks) and *ludus* ('fun' but also 'school'—*ludus schola*—for the Romans).

According to Plato, to be educational, play involving children had to: favour movement, be done in a group—in a place consecrated to the gods—mix males and females and be supervised by nursemaids to moderate the liveliness. Furthermore, it also must have a set of fixed rules, which make it possible to test and specify the socialisation processes. This is a very modern attitude, and within the experimentation of these mutual relationships among play participants lies the possibility of moral growth.

Basically, however, in ancient times, educational attention on play focused mainly on the development of gymnastic and sport skills and to prepare for war.[38]

In the Middle Ages, it was the Church that provided a strong orientation regarding the area of play, that was considered an activity to be controlled, since it was a possible source of moral promiscuity and some games may be dangerous for moral development;[39] play was kept under control: if on one hand, it was necessary to educate, on the other, it was necessary to allow to vent itself because—as Fénelon asserts—children have their own innate 'great heat'.

Locke's idea of play can be considered a precursor of modern pedagogy; according to him, toys must not be purchased, but made by the children themselves: "little stones, a pack of cards, a mother's keys, and other similar items that they can't hurt themselves with are fun for children just as much as those things that are bought at such a dear price in stores and that go bad or break in a very short time" (Locke, 1918, orig. ed. 1693). Study should be just as fun as play, and if a child wants to continue

37 This paragraph is largely inspired by Besio (2008).

38 In more modern times, motor play has been studied mainly by Parlebas (1990), who emphasised its relationship with specific cultural models, including rules (e.g., the game of tag). It combines affectivity and the fantasies of the child and not only the motor coordination abilities, and is capable of reaching conscious and unconscious levels. Comparative studies have been developed between different types of games, such as football and baseball, about how they are structured from a motor viewpoint, the role that they identify, the type of relationships that they suggest and create, and not only because of their rules.

39 Around the 1400s, distinguishing features were making headway within the general attitude of condemnation: there was a focus on ludus licitus, ludus tolerabilis, ludus indifferens, ludus ricreation, up to ludus laudabilis that consists of the holy representations of the life of saints.

to play, it's a sign that he or she is not yet ready to study. There is a pedagogical advantage in the efforts children make while playing: "I thus thought that if games were invented with a certain contrivance it would be possible to find many ways to teach kids to read in a way that would seem almost like playing to them" (Locke, cit.).

For Fénelon (cit.), play can be functional to the needs of education, making study more pleasurable—"let's hide study behind the appearance of freedom and pleasure"—then from games, we must remove everything that can make children overly excited, or that permits the simultaneous presence of males and females: in other words, play can make you lose your head or can be a source of sinful thoughts.[40]

The era of Illuminism represents the great turning point in the European history regarding education, because pedagogy put the focus on creating citizens and disseminating social values. The educational process must move towards the illuminist project of citizens, who must not only understand and adapt to laws, but be possibly capable of developing new ones.

The educational utility of play is clearer at this point: Basedow (1914, orig. ed. 1768) was the first to knowingly link play with educational activity, for example, inventing school competitions—and many linguistic ones—in which children could try to beat the other peers in the group and with which they could have a lot of fun; and fun—conceived in this case mainly as a joke—was an integral part of the education project through play.

However, it is only with Fröbel (1967, orig. ed. 1826) that play acquires its full educational value: it stimulates the imagination and allows the child to relate with himself or herself and with the world. To carry out these functions, play cannot be solitary, but with a group, and must allow children to practice skills and roles that they can adopt and do as adults. As known, Fröbel invented the mechanism of 'gifts' to offer to children to favour their growth that is seen as total, of body and mind ("the body and its parts must be made capable of obeying the spirit at any time"), growth that must take place at the same pace, following the same path (Provenzo, 2009). Thus, recreational education requires particular attention: movement and play must be developed together and gradually at different ages. Physical strength and moral and spiritual determination exist in a direct relationship that, through play, can be taught. He encouraged children to engage in self-directed manipulations of the material world, so that they can join scientific knowledge with an aesthetic experience (Henricks, 2014).

Fröbel's educational project is based on some fundamental features that are still quite interesting: a) play is a planned part of the school day; the adult must not act

40 Piaget himself was interested in play as the source of moral thought, because it leads to awareness of moral relationships in society: :The individual by himself remains egocentric. The solution lies in a comparison among children, in their playing and working together, in the negotiation of meanings and rules and in cooperation" (Piaget, 1980, orig. ed. 1932).

in an authoritative manner; b) the use of structured educational materials that carry out the explicit function of teachings; c) play must be correlated to the environment in which it is carried out and be open to contact with nature; d) the creative and cognitive aspects present in play must be safeguarded and nurtured at the same time; e) the link between play and life is explicit; the recreational behaviour can become a social behaviour.

Since Fröbel opened history's first kindergarten in 1837 and wrote that play is the highest phase of child development, incorporating play into early childhood programmes has almost been synonymous with the pedagogy of the field. The progressive school educator of the first quarter of the 20th century then built upon Fröbel's emphasis on the importance of play.

Then, Maria Montessori's (1936; 1949) famous method encourages children to play with elements that have implications for adult life, such as toy hammers, dishes, and ovens. According to her, children desire self-guided activity with culturally valued items instead of fantasy-based role play; they also enjoy the social validation that comes from sharing their activities with peers. The entire educational system of Montessori is based on the seriousness of adult work. The play impulse in children is really a work impulse; its two main characteristics—the tendency to be active and the tendency to be experimental—can be assets of education.

For Dewey (1910), the relationship with materials is of great importance: materials are seen as real tools, if the situation is governed by playful spirit, which commits them to the inherent value of what they are doing and excites their creativity. The value of play was greatly emphasised, as something that builds the person, through experiences but also by habits of self-directed enquiry: "In short, the grounds for assigning play a definite place in the curriculum are intellectual and social not matters of temporary expediency and momentary agreeableness. Without something of the kind, it is not possible to secure the normal estate of effective learning; namely, that knowledge-getting be an outgrowth of activities having their own end instead of a school task" (1944:195).

Also, to Piaget, play is a way to engage children in the learning process: "This is why play is such a powerful lever in the learning process of very young children and to such an extent that whenever anyone can succeed in transforming their first steps in reading, arithmetic or spelling into a game, you will see they become passionately absorbed in these occupations which are ordinarily presented as dreary chores" (Piaget, 1972:155).

The consequences of adopting play in the educational process are, for Vygotskij, not so subservient to fragmented aspects of learning, but rather related to the child's development 'per se', as play is a leading factor in development: "Children's great achievements are possible in play, achievements that tomorrow will become their basic level of real action and morality" (Vygotskij, 1978:100).

1.5.2 The Difficult Relationship Between Play and Education: Controlling Play[41]

Where does the relationship between infant play activity and learning begin? Is it possible to have fun while learning? Can teaching be made fun? And, is it beneficial to make learning fun? What is the difference between play in other contexts and play in educational contexts? Is it possible to teach how to play, without having in mind teaching something other than play?

In what follows, an attempt is made to track the most important steps of the relationship between play and education, which has been more controversial than what might be expected; and it is still in this way.

Generally speaking, the scholastic context can take advantage of the instructional-educational values shared with play: in fact, it has the ability to positively interfere with the child's growth factors identified as always as pedagogic objectives.

- *Cognitive* development a) increases the mental reprocessing of reality (abstraction, imagination, fantasy); b) favours the exploration of the world of possibilities and hypotheses; c) develops creative and inventive skills and decentralisation capacities through symbolic play; d) requires the adoption and experimentation of *planning* and *problem-solving* strategies.
- *Emotive-affective* development permits and develops: a) the expression and control of emotions; b) a realistic awareness of self; c) personal independence.
- *Socio-relational skills* favour: a) respect for the rules; b) ability to cooperate; c) ability to mediate and negotiate.
- *Socio-cognitive* development (Ashman & Conway, 1989; Bandura, 2001) influences structuring and consolidation of a) motivation; b) self-efficiency; c) self-esteem; d) prosociality; e) agentivity.

As seen in the previous paragraph, 'historic' pedagogy has focused on the value and role of play in education and considers it as a learning mediator, even when it was bestowed the role of a protagonist; it is since the first years of the 1900s that play became a significant part of the early childhood school curriculum.

In the contemporary literature of the field, there is a greater awareness, which corresponds to an important amount of studies, about the role of play as the main

41 The study of the role that play has taken in time in the pedagogical field, and above all, that it has now in education, forms the basis for reflecting on the role that play has for the education of children with disabilities. It should not be forgotten anyway that children with disabilities spend most of their time in rehabilitation activities and settings. The relationship between education and the rehabilitation frameworks has not been addressed clearly until now; what is clear enough is that both—education and rehabilitation—aim for the same goal: give the child an opportunity to make positive and useful experiences, for training new effective abilities, so positively influencing the structure of the brain and consolidating new learning. This possibility is recently supported and deepened by neuroscience studies (Sandman & Kemp, 2007).

activity of the developing child, as well as a more clear consciousness about the different types of educational settings—formal, informal, non-formal[42]—with which the child comes into contact. Moreover, one could say that for each of the different functions of play highlighted by scholars, there is an educational-didactic or rehabilitative-therapeutical application: so, play can become a tool to foster learning, the privileged means to encourage socialisation, and to promote the expression of feelings as well as their control, while in some cases, it becomes the main road to get into the child's inner world, providing an instrument for cure and assessment.

1.5.2.1 Play and Play-like Activities

Inevitably, however, all these interpretations and uses of play are, to some extent, dominated by the objective for which the play activity is proposed and programmed; while play has extraordinary educational value and can be used as an incomparable educational 'hook', it undoubtedly loses some of its play features: for example, freedom, pure ludic spirit, transgression, autonomous initiative, and autotelism.

It was the Italian pedagogist Aldo Visalberghi (1958) who systematised these issues clearly, in a way that is still productive today for a critical reading of the existing research in the field and for future directions. Indeed, according to him, the play activity has the following characteristics: a) it is *demanding*, it requires a complete commitment by the player;[43] b) it is *continuative*, it develops continuously in a child's life;[44] c) it is *progressive*, because it can become gradually and increasingly complex; no play activity is exclusively repetitive and equal to itself;[45] d) it envisages the *end* of an activity, not requiring a continuation once the game has ended.[46]

Many activities carried out in schools or in educational contexts that include learning objectives can have the appearance and even the structure of play activities and can, of course, have amusing and fun characteristics. For these activities and programmes, Visalberghi proposes the expression *play-like*. They have the same

42 According to OECD (2010): a) *formal* learning is always organised and structured, and has learning objectives; from the learner's standpoint, it is always intentional; b) *informal* learning is never organised, has no set objective in terms of learning outcomes, and is never intentional from the learner's standpoint; often it is referred to as learning by experience or just as experience; c) *non-formal* learning is rather organised and can have learning objectives. Such learning may occur at the initiative of the individual, but also happens as a byproduct of more organised activities, whether or not the activities themselves have learning objectives.

43 This point can be considered in analogy with the characteristics of commitment, intrinsic motivation, and intensity, but also with the fundamental of doing, which creates and requires continuous challenges.

44 This theme can be connected with the evolutivity of play and with its characteristic of freedom that permeates it entirely.

45 This aspect can be seen in relation to the fundamental of evolutivity of play and with its characteristic of flexibility.

46 This argument is directly associated with 'being in play', the in-lusio and the framework of Bateson.

first three characteristics as the play activities, but not the fourth one, since they do not end in themselves, but have educational objectives and a final scope, that of learning.

Play-like activities and educational games are an integral part of the educational life and process, which start from nursery school, and according to Scurati, can be found also in the play-like games of pre-adolescence, which must be understood as an authentically autotelic event (or as a phenomenon that has in itself its own scope) and "as a mere hetero-formative device, understood as a kind of sophisticated adultistic camouflage, a trick device" (Scurati, 2000, cited in Besio, 2008:23). In fact, in this case, the intentionality of giving cultural contents would be so open as to impede the real involvement of the learner, preventing him or her from getting into the play atmosphere.

Useful signals indicating that one is in a context of 'controlled playfulness' or 'goal-oriented playfulness' are given by: well-structured relational rapports, presence of expressed rules, and a stable guide provided by adults or educators who, in fact, are familiar with and declare the end of the activity, and thus define its times and procedures.

In these cases, the adult or educator can also act as a mediator between the relationships of children to modulate the complexity of the game so that it will match the varying level of capacities of each person, to guide the movement of the activity if necessary by referring to the defined rules, and so on. Examples of play-like activities and programmes can be:

a) Activities intentionally created and materials expressly used to give a fun and pleasant form to certain types of learning actions that are considered complex—thus requiring special concentration and reasoning—or boring because of their repetitive nature (e.g. games such as domino or bingo to learn multiplication tables; nursery rhymes to learn automatic series such as the alphabet or the months of the year; attractive and fun toys to support the accomplishment of psychomotor or cognitive activities that would be difficult otherwise).
b) Learning contexts[47] and programmes proposed to groups of children—but also to individuals—informed in a playful manner, so that the educational objectives are part of the play situation itself even if they remain extrinsic to play (e.g., symbolic play sessions proposed to develop the pragmatic aspects of verbal language or to monitor the concomitant development of other symbolic competences; construction play planned to test the child's memory span or competence in operating the technical aspects of building with blocks—dimensions, weights, and so on—practice play in the playground designed to verify and improve the child's psychomotor abilities or balance); in other words, the play situation becomes the best way to convey and pursue the educational objective, in any field it belongs.

47 For different contexts of learning, see also Note 38.

c) Learning contexts and programmes created for the purpose of giving the group of children the possibility to explore and actively adopt co-operative approaches and techniques in working and playing together; social competence is mainly addressed in this case for creating worthy societies: “play is inquiry into the challenges and responsibilities of social living” (Henricks, 2015:4).

Today, the commitment to play can be found in early childhood programmes in many different countries (Wood & Artfield, 2005). “Many programs today organize the space, materials and time of the curriculum around a focus on children’s play (Frost et al., 2005; Sluss, 2005). The space of the modern classroom is divided and arranged into activity areas or centres, defining the type of play that will occur within the particular space of the classroom. These areas or centres are then stocked with the materials needed to support the type of play that is to occur. The typical daily schedule of early childhood programs now also provides a designated amount of time for play, often labelled free play time, activity time or choice time. In most cases, this is a time of the day during which children are free to choose the area or centre in which they want to play, and once there they are free to choose what they do with the materials available for them in that area” (Kuschner, 2015:288-289).

Adopting Visalberghi’s systematisation, we could say that on the one hand, play-like activities and contexts have taken the field and spread at least in the young child’s education, while the space of play as such has been transferred and included into the denomination ‘free play’: during free play time, the child is left free to do what he or she wants, but this somehow weakens the play’s educational value, because it is only considered as a free outburst (Bredekamp, 2004).[48]

48 An examination of the contemporary relationship between play and early childhood education reveals, however, a paradoxical tension: “On the one hand, children’s play has long been regarded as strengthening the fabric of early childhood education at child-care centers, nursery schools, preschools, kindergartens, and the first three grades of elementary schools. Yet on the other hand, educators of children between the ages of three to seven have sharply contested how to weave play into classroom practice. And further, many schools now shrink from play” (Kuschner, 2015:287). The disagreements and tensions concerning play and early childhood education are still with us today, especially in Northern European countries; it has been noted that “in recent years, children’s play has come under serious attack. Many preschools and elementary schools have reduced or even eliminated playtime from their schedules” (Zigler & Bishop-Joseph, 2004:1). It seems that didactic instruction and testing are pushing play out of the kindergarten; most forms of schooling or education are “less interested in what comes out of the child than they are in what can be put into or transmitted to the child” (Kuschner, 2015:287). Thus, as children play is “not just in response to external stimuli but also in accord with internal ideas” (Berk, 1994:32), they become less curious about play. Kindergartens are now under intense pressure to meet inappropriate expectations, including academic standards. These expectations and policies that result from them have greatly reduced, and in some cases, obliterated opportunities for imaginative child initiated play in kindergarten.

1.5.2.2 The Role of Adults in Supporting a Child's Play

Two aspects of the play-curriculum relationship have been addressed within the research on play in the context of early childhood education. Within these studies, play is primarily viewed as a means to foster child development in disciplinary domains. They also gave rise to practical suggestions on "how to create math- or literacy-rich play environments and on how to incorporate math, science or literacy language into children's play (Van Oers & Wardekker, 1999)" (Bodrova & Leong, 2010:2).[49]

Another line of play research has been done in naturalistic settings with children engaged in free play with little or no adult guidance; it focusses on the multiple forms that play might assume (e.g., social, pretend, or object), stressing the fact that it is like a child-initiated activity; "these contributions are associated with the development of broader competencies such as theory of mind (Berk et al., 2006), symbolic representation (Rogers & Evans: 2007), and self-regulation (Miller & Almon, 2009) that not only affect child development in early years but have a long-lasting effect in the school years and beyond" (Bodrova & Leong, 2010:2).

Recommendations for the curriculum coming from these studies emphasise both "the provision of adequate physical spaces and props to support play" and "the need to allow ample time for children's free play in the preschool daily schedule and preserve or increase recess time for kindergartners and children in the primary grades (Farran & Son-Yarbrough, 2001; Smirnova & Gudareva, 2004)" (Bodrova & Leong 2010:2).

This clear separation between the study of play in educational settings and for educational goals from one hand and the study of free play and of its possible developmental consequences on the other is also affected by what Wood (2008) calls "ideological commitment to free play and free choice".

This has, however, largely lost sight of the substantial role of the adult within the playful situations; in field studies, "while there is substantial evidence on learning through play, there is less evidence on teaching through play" (Wood, 2009:27). The focus should, on the contrary, shift to better understanding the distinctive purposes and nature of play in educational settings and the role of adults in planning for play and playfulness in child-initiated or teacher-directed activities.

The pedagogy of play "is defined broadly as the ways in which early childhood professionals make provision for play and playful approaches to learning and

49 "One set of researchers look into the use of play elements, play environments, or play motivation as a way to enhance instruction in core subjects such as literacy (Saracho & Spodek, 2006; Ginsburg, 2006), mathematics (Fleer, 2009; Uren & Stagnitti, 2009) or science (Dickinson, 2001), or as a way to promote specific areas of development such as the development of children's social-emotional competencies (Connor et al., 2006), oral language (Pellegrini 2009; Pullen & Justice 2003) or gross and fine motor skills (Lillard, 2001), etc." (Bodrova & Leong 2010:1).

teaching, how they design play/learning environments, and all the pedagogical decisions, techniques and strategies they use to support or enhance learning and teaching through play" (Wood, 2009:27).

However, the importance of home-based pedagogies of play and the ways in which children teach themselves how to play during their self-initiated activities should not be underestimated. According to an English large-scale longitudinal study,[50] which explored the specific pedagogical actions linking play with positive learning outcomes (Sylva et al., 2007), it is necessary to distinguish between "pedagogical interactions (specific behaviours on the part of adults) and pedagogical framing (the behind-the-scenes aspects of pedagogy which include planning resources and routines)" (Wood, 2009:29). According to the Effective Provision of Pre-School Education (EPPE) scholars, "the most effective (excellent) settings provide both and achieve a balance between the opportunities provided for children to benefit from teacher-initiated group work and the provision of freely chosen yet potentially instructive play activities" (EPPE, 2002:43).

"Indicators of effective pedagogy include opportunities for co-construction between children and adults, including 'sustained shared thinking', joint involvement in child and adult-initiated activities and informed interactions in children's self-initiated and free-play activities. The practitioner's role is conceptualized as proactive in creating play/learning environments, as well as responsive to children's choices, interests and patterns of learning" (Wood, 2009:29).

This means that learning through play should not be left to improvisation nor to incident; pedagogical models should be developed and adopted for sustaining 'complex and reciprocal relationships' and organising 'socially constructed and mediated' activities; play should be 'endorsed within integrated pedagogical approaches', but the current situation is not homogeneous all over the world. While in the UK, for example, achieving good-quality play in practice remains a considerable challenge, as teachers face competing demands for accountability, performance and achievement, the experience of the Reggio Children school model in Italy has been acclaimed worldwide for being significant. Teachers and children are here engaged, together with families, in applying and developing an educational model based on participation, observation, mediation, and discussion, according to the constructivist approach. "The physical environment (the 'amiable' school) receives much attention and supports exchange and relationships through physical qualities of transparency, reflectiveness, openness, harmony, softness, and light (Ceppi & Zini, 1998; Gandini, 1993). A classroom atmosphere of playfulness and joy pervades. The school and surrounding community welcome the children into

50 The study, conducted in the UK in 2004 and named EPPE (Effective Provision for Preschool Education; www.ioe.ac.uk/RB_Final_Report_3-7.pdf) "has provided detailed evidence of the impact of preschool education and family background on children's development" (Wood, 2009:28).

their culture and toward democratic participation" (Pope Edwards, 2002:9). Play is here considered a source of identity, imagination, freedom; this "makes the idea of play as freedom a natural assumption in the Reggio experience. The will of an individual, if fully nourished and multilaterally expressed within a community, is regarded as a positive and creative force. With the folk memory of totalitarianism lingering in the Reggio consciousness, this makes the 'right to play' more than just a fashionable assertion" (Kane, 2004:282-283).

1.5.2.3 Need for Clarity: Roles, Terminology, Activities

These reflections help to understand the level of awareness the debate on play and education reached, though with some contrasts, in recent decades.

The use of play for educational purposes—or rather, the organisation of ludic activities and programmes that directly influence the educational and developmental levels—made it possible to state useful considerations about the role of the adults in play, on how their collaboration can be less directive, more collaborative, more available to listen to the child's playful initiative, which is instead usually left to a phase of free play, for which the adults decide not to participate. Furthermore, the convincing results of ad hoc research projects made it possible to contrast that 'ideological commitment' that wanted to preserve a certain idea of 'freedom' in play, according to which its introduction in educational settings, or even the participation of adults, eventually pollute its natural evolution and inherent creativity, even influencing a child's development.

According to a research by Bennet et al. (1997), "where children follow their own interests and agendas the teachers realize the need to understand the meaning of play in children's own terms, rather than in relation to predetermined learning objectives. [...] In particular, they realized that children need more time to develop sustained bouts of play, and to return to their own themes and ongoing interests" (Wood, 2009:30).

"Miller and Almon (2009) recommend that neither laissez-faire free play nor didactic highly structured classrooms are the answer, but rather classrooms that are rich in child-initiated play and activities initiated playfully by teachers. They believe that young children need a balance of child-initiated play and more structured and focused experiential learning activities, all occurring in the presence of skilled and engaged teachers" (Kuschner, 2015:289).

"However, the lack of a common definition of play makes it hard to provide specific recommendations for curriculum designers and to advocate for preserving play in early childhood classrooms in the face of increasing demands for a focus on academic skills. One way to solve this dilemma is to use more specific terms like 'playful learning' to make a distinction between child initiated play and adult-initiated activities that make use of play elements in one form or another. This may help to avoid confusions that lead to certain curricula to be labelled as 'play-based' when in reality they leave no time for children to initiate play on their own. However, the distinction between play and playful learning has to be made clear both in the description of their objectives and the specific pedagogies associated with each of them. In addition, this also calls for more in-depth analysis of how exactly play elements are used in instruction and whether their use is perceived as 'playful' by children themselves or only by the teachers" (Bodrova & Leong, 2009:3).

So, interesting and promising studies and researches are starting, aimed at achieving greater pedagogical awareness in educators, practitioners, if possible in adults 'tout court', about specific modes of interaction and cooperation to be adopted within the play framework and activity, in order to promote the child's development in certain areas.

Among these, some proposals try to establish connections between the children and their teachers, with regard to their attitude about play. In support of the idea that the dichotomy between learning and play is a false one, researchers of NAEYC[51] argue that both direct instruction and play have roles in high-quality early childhood education. Some studies compared children's behaviour when provided with direct instruction (of a sort) about how to activate a novel toy, and when allowed to explore the toy without explicit instruction (a sort of free-play condition). Both children given direct instruction and children in the free play mode learnt the intended use of the toy, but the latter also discovered additional uses of the toy or its pieces; only this group of children showed creativity and problem-solving skills not necessary in the direct instruction condition (Hirsh-Paseck et al., 2009). After the publication of these studies, Snow (2011) proposed that a new strategy to find "the middle ground between play and direct instruction is to view instruction and play as two ways of defining activity in classrooms" (Figure 1.1.). In it, the degrees of child activity and teacher activity are mapped onto each other. The resulting four quadrants show the overlap between teacher instructional strategies (as more or less actively directing) and child play activities. Both of these approaches challenge us to think about the roles of teacher and child, and of play and instruction, in more complex and more intentional ways.

51 It is the acronym of the US National Association for the Education of Young Children, www.naeyc.org.

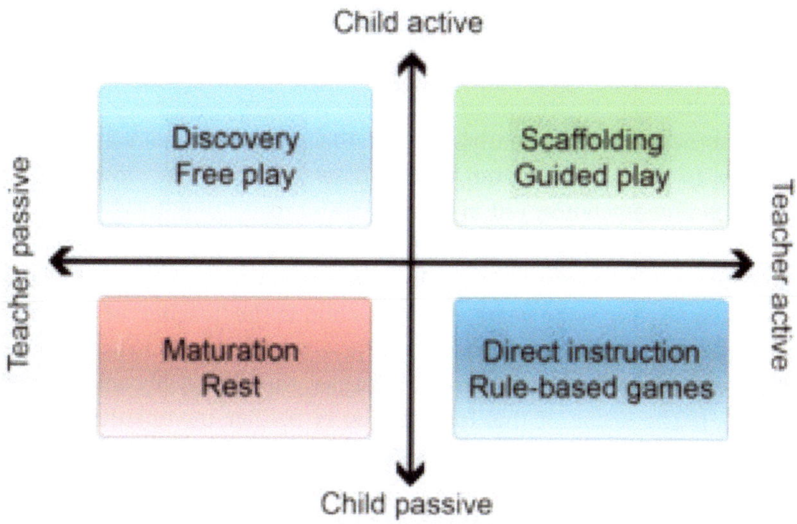

Figure 1.1. Instructed and free play: relationships between teachers and children (Snow, 2011)

1.5.2.4 Play for the Sake of Play

It must be said, however, that these considerations are mainly related, rather than to play itself, to play-like activities and contexts: activities and contexts of play based on programmatically clear educational goals, demanding not only precise planning, but also a different and more complex, participation of the adult.

There is an additional area of reflection and analysis that until now has been overlooked, and is the subject of the development of play as such, for the purpose and objectives of the play itself: what in this section has been called 'play for the sake of play'.

Play, as we have seen, cannot have extrinsic preordained goals—it lives, arises, develops, and stops, only for itself; it is free, but not without limits, and indeed seeks out and constructs by itself the constraint to become more exciting, compelling, and challenging. It resorts to the use of routines and requires rapid changes, evolving towards new and more promising types, and then intertwining the new types with the previous ones, that are already known.

It definitely 'produces' learning on a large scale and in many areas of the individual's development, but it never patently pursues such a purpose. While playing with adults, a child shows play levels of greater complexity and appears more concentrated; this also happens in the case of play with more experienced peers—even if to a different extent and in different ways. These play relationships activate the proximal zone of development.

Play for the sake of play can also be learnt. An educator or a practitioner can enter the child's play to improve, increase, and develop it. not for reaching external goals, not to turn it into a play-like activity, but only to pursue objectives inherent to the play itself.

This awareness is not yet clearly shared in the field sciences: it's about learning to enter play, to play with children, with full awareness of one's own adulthood and educational competence, but maintaining and respecting the constraints and limitations of play itself and taking action to consolidate it, change it, and increase its complexity and flexibility as play, not as a means of learning or development. Bondioli noted already some years ago: "the child is the 'teacher' of play and the adult who plays with the child should not have other intention than play itself, neither to instruct, nor to train. It is a 'negative' role which becomes a positive behaviour [...]. The scope of this ludic action is neither therapeutic nor strictly 'educational', but simply ludic: happy sharing is simultaneously its meaning and its purpose" (Bondioli, 2002:86).

The adult who plays with a child shares his or her own ludic experience with that child, and this interaction will become more advantageous the more the adult's infancy has been richly, extensively, and broadly playful. Playing with a child also means losing the typical adult/child asymmetry, becoming immersed in reciprocity and sharing. It is also a form of sentimental education as it paves the way to listening to the infant's innerness, sharing the emotional reality that appears in play.

This can only be achieved if the adult has in mind a clear developmental model of play, to sustain the child's action, and to 'work with and through play': its characteristics, its mechanisms, its rhythms, its times and needs. In other words, the adult would greatly benefit of having in mind the evolutionary spiral on which any type of play is grafted, as well as the need to indulge both unpredictability and rigorousness.

It is not a simple goal to achieve, and probably, specific training will be needed. In fact, "teachers and practitioners strive to constrain and manage the unpredictability of play that is truly free and aim instead to engineer children's play choices and behaviours in ways that promote educational outcomes. And, if play is to be purposeful, then whose purposes are privileged, and whose purposes are being served: those of the child, the practitioners or the curriculum?" (Wood, 2009:32).

Practitioners need to understand better and more deeply the meaning of children's play activities, and they should know and adopt the appropriate scaffolding strategies to support the interactions between children and between the child and the adult. They should also become more aware of how to plan the educational curricula in order to combine activities that are directed by themselves and those that are initiated by the children. "These integrated approaches require high levels of pedagogical knowledge and skills, flexibility in curriculum planning assessment and evaluation" (Wood, 2009:33).

According to Wood, "further conceptual advances can be facilitated through socio-cultural and activity theories which propose that play is a social practice and is situated in communities of practice" (ibidem). If learning is socially mediated and constructed within an everyday 'real world' mixed with the 'play world', "play activities may facilitate the transfer of knowledge across different contexts, with the distinction that play occurs in imagined situations. Players become part of a discourse community in which meanings, intentions and activities are communicated through mediating means: imagined situations, tools, symbolic actions, scripts, roles and rules" (ibidem).

In this sense, play also becomes the privileged means for creating inclusive contexts and adopting inclusive styles, with respect to any kind of differences, including those related to the possible impairments and to human functioning.

References

Ashman, A. F., & Conway, R. N. F. (1989). *Cognitive strategies for special education*. London, UK: Routledge.

Avedon, E. M., & Sutton-Smith, B. (1971). *The Study of Games*. New York, NY: John Wiley & Sons.

Bandura, A. (2001). Social cognitive theory. An agentic perspective. *Annual Review of Psychology*, 52, 1-26.

Bateson, G. (1956). *The Message "This Is Play"*. Princeton, NJ: Josia Macy Jr. Foundation.

Bateson, G. (1972). *Steps to an Ecology of Mind*. Chicago, IL: The University of Chicago Press.

Bennett, N. L., Wood, L., & Rogers, S. (1997). Teaching through play: Teachers' thinking and classroom practice. Buckingham, UK: Open University Press.

Berk, L. E. (1994). Vygotskij's theory: The importance of make believe. *Young children*, 50, 1, 30-39.

Berk, L.E., Mann, T.D., & Ogan. A.T. (2006). *Make-believe play: Wellspring for development of self-regulation*. In: D. G. Singer, R. M. Golinkoff, & K. Hirsh-Pasek (Eds.), *Play = Learning: How play motivates and enhances children's cognitive and social-emotional growth* (pp. 74-100). New York, NY: Oxford University Press.

Besio, S. (2008). *Analysis of Critical Factors Involved in using interactive Robots for Education and Therapy of children with disabilities*. Trento, I: Uniservice.

Bettelheim, B. (1972). Play and education. *School Review*, 819, 1-13.

Bettelheim, B. (1984). The importance of play. *Atlantic Monthly*, March, 35-46.

Bodrova, E., & Leong, D.J. (2010). Curriculum and Play. *Encyclopedia on Early Childhood Development. CEECD / SKC-ECD.*

Bodrova, E., & Leong, D. J. (2015). Standing "A Head Taller Than Himself": Vygotskian and Post-Vygotskian Views on Children's Play. In: J. E. Johnson, S. G. Eberle, T. S. Henricks, & D. Kuschne (Eds.), *The Handbook of the Study of Play* (pp. 203-214). Lanham, MD: Rowman & Littlefield Publishing Group.

Bondioli, A. (2002). *Gioco e educazione* [Play and education]. Milano, I: Franco Angeli.

Bredekamp, S. (2004). *Play and school readiness*. In: E. Zigler, D. Singer, & S. Bishop-Josef (Eds.), *Children's play: The roots of reading* (pp. 159-174). Washington, D.C.: Zero to Three Press.

Broadhead, P. (2004). *Early Years Play and Learning: Developing Social Skills and Co-operation*. London, UK: Routledge Falmer.

Bruner, J.S. (1986). *Actual Minds, Possible Worlds*. Cambridge, MA: Harvard University Press.

Bundy, A. C. (1993). Assessment of play and leisure. Delineation of the problem. *The American Journal of Occupational Therapy*, 47(3), 217-222.

Bundy, A. C. (2000). *Test of Playfulness (Revised version 3.5) manual*. Ft. Collins, CO: Colorado State University.

Bundy, A.C., Nelson, L., Metzger, M., & Bingaman, K. (2001). Validity and reliability of the Test of Playfulness. *Occupational Therapy Journal of Research*, 21, 276-292.

Caillois, R. (2001). *Les jeux et les hommes*. Paris, F: Gallimard (or. ed., 1958).

Caillois, R. (1967). *Jeux et sports*. Paris, F: Gallimard.

Ceppi, G., & Zini, M. (1998). *Children, spaces, relations: Metaproject for an environment for young children*. Reggio Emilia, I: Municipality of Reggio Emila Infanzia Ricerca.

Clements R. D., & Fiorentino, L. (2004). *The Child's Right to Play: A Global Approach*. Westport, CT. Praeger Publishers.

Connor, C. M., Morrison, F. L., & Slominski, L. (2006). Preschool instruction and children's emergent literacy growth. *Journal of Educational Psychology*, 98(4), 665- 689.

Coplan, R. J., Ooi, L. L., Kirkpatrick, A., & Rubin, K. H. (2015). *Social and Nonsocial Play*. In: D. Bergen, & D. Fromberg (Eds.), *Play from Birth to Twelve and Beyond: Contexts, Perspectives, and Meanings* (pp. 97-106). New York & London: Garland Publishing.

Csikszentmihalyi, M. (1990). *Flow: The psychology of optimal experience*. New York, NY: Harper & Row.

Csikszentmihalyi, M. (1997). *Finding flow. The psychology of engagement in everyday life*. New York, NY: Basic Books.

De Lisi, R. (2015). Piaget's Sympathetic But Unromantic Account of Children's Play. In: J. E. Johnson, S. G. Eberle, T. S. Henricks, & D. Kuschne (Eds), *The Handbook of the Study of Play* (pp. 227-238). Lanham, MD: Rowman & Littlefield Publishing Group.

Dewey, J. (1944). *Democracy and Education*. New York, NY: Macmillan (or. ed., 1944).

Dickinson, D. K. (2001). Large-group and free-play times: Conversational settings supporting language and literacy development. In: D. K. Dickinson, & P. O. Tabors (Eds.), *Beginning literacy with language: Young children learning at home and school* (pp. 223–256). Baltimore, MD: Paul H. Brookes Publishing.

Eberle, S. G. (2014). The Elements of Play Toward a Philosophy and a Definition of Play. *Journal of Play*, 6(2), 214-233.

Ellis, M. (1973). *Why people play*. Englewood Cliffs, NJ: Prentice-Hall.

Erickson, E. (1963). *Childhood and Society*. New York, NY: Norton.

Farran, D., & Son-Yarbrough, W. (2001). I funded preschools as a developmental context for children's play and verbal behaviors. *Early Childhood Research Quarterly*, 16(2), 245-262.

Fein, G. G. (1981). Pretend Play in Childhood: An Integrative Review. *Child Development*, 52, 1095-1118.

Fein, G. G. (1987). Pretend Play: Creativity and Consciousness. In: D. Gorlitz, & J. F. Wohlwill (Eds.), *Curiosity, imagination and play: On the development of spontaneous cognitive and motivational processes* (pp. 282-304). Hillsdale, NJ: Erlbaum.

Fink, E. (1986). *Oasi della gioia. Idee per una ontologia del gioco* [Oasis of joy. Ideas for an ontology of play]. Salerno, I: Masullo (orig. ed., *Oase des Glücks. Gedanken zu einer Ontologie des Spiels*, 1957).

Fink, E. (1992). *Il gioco come simbolo del mondo* [Play as symbol of the world]. Firenze, I: Hopeful Monster (or. ed., *Spiel als Weltsymbol*, 1960).

Fleer, M. (2009). Supporting scientific conceptual consciousness or learning in a roundabout way in play-based contexts. *International Journal of Science Education*, 31(8), 1069-1089.

Fornari, F. (1988). *La vita affettiva originaria del bambino* [Child's early affective life]. Milano, I: Feltrinelli (or. ed., 1963).

Freud, S. (1977). *Al di là del principio di piacere* [Beyond the pleasure principle]. Torino, I: Boringhieri (or. ed., *Jenseits des Lustprinzips*, 1920).

Frost, J. L., Wortham, S. C., & Reifel, S. (2005). *Play and child development*. Upper Saddle River, NJ: Prentice Hall.

Gandini, L. (1993). *Fundamentals of the Reggio Emilia approach to early childhood education*. Young Children, 49(1), 4-8.

Garner, B. P., & Bergen, D. (2015). Play Development from Birth to Age Four. In: D. Bergen, & D. Fromberg (Eds.), *Play from Birth to Twelve and Beyond: Contexts, Perspectives, and Meanings* (pp. 11-20). New York & London: Garland Publishing.

Garvey, C. (1976). Some properties of social play. In: J.S. Bruner, A. Jolly, & K. Silva (Eds.), *Play. Its role in Development and Evolution* (pp. 570-584). New York, NY: Basic Books.

Garvey, C. (1982). Communication and the development of social role play. In: D. Forbes, & M.T. Greenberg (Eds). *New directions for child development. No. 18. Children's planning strategies*. San Francisco, CA: Jossey-Bass.

Garvey, C. (1990). *Play*. Cambridge, MA: Harvard University Press.

Geertz, C. (1973). *The Interpretation of Cultures*. New York, NY: Basic Books.

Gily, C. (2006). *In-lusio. Il gioco come formazione estetica*. Napoli, I: Scriptaweb.

Ginsburg, H. P. (2006). Mathematical play and playful mathematics: A guide for early education. In: D. G. Singer, R. M. Golinkoff, & K. Hirsh-Pasek (Eds.), *Play = Learning: How play motivates and enhances children's cognitive and social-emotional growth* (pp. 145-165). New York, NY: Oxford University Press.

Goncü, A., & Gaskins, S. (2011). Comparing and extending Piaget's and Vygotskij's understanding of play: Symbolic play as individual, sociocultural and educational interpretation. In. A.D. Pellegrini (Ed.), *The Oxford Handbook of the Development of Play* (pp. 48-57). New York, NY: Oxford University Press

Gordon, G. (2009). What Is Play? In Search of a Definition. In: D. Kuschner (Ed.), *From Children to Red Hatters: Diverse Images and Issues of Play* (pp. 1-13). Lanham, MD: United Press of America.

Groos, K. (1901). *The Play of Man*. New York, NY: Appleton.

Haight, W. (1998). Adult direct and indirect influences on play. In: D. Bergen, D. Fromberg (Eds.), *Play from Birth to Twelve and Beyond: Contexts, Perspectives, and Meanings* (pp. 259-265). New York & London: Garland Publishing.

Haight, W. (2015). A Sociocultural Perspective of Parent-Child Play. In: D. Bergen, D. Fromberg (Eds.), *Play from Birth to Twelve and Beyond: Contexts, Perspectives, and Meanings* (pp. 309-314). New York, NY: Routledge

Harding, J., Meldon-Smith, L., & Sheridan, M. (2012). *Play in Early Childhood: From Birth to Six Years*. London, UK and New York, NY: Routledge.

Henricks, T.S. (2009). *Play and the Rhetorics of Time: Progress, Regression, and the Meaning of the Present*. In: D. Kuschner (Ed.), *From Children to Red Hatters: Diverse Images and Issues of Play* (pp. 14-38). Lanham: United Press of America.

Henricks, T. S. (2014). Play as Self-Realization. Toward a General Theory of Play. *American Journal of Play*, 6, 2, 190-213.

Henricks, T. S. (2015). *Sociological Perspectives on Play*. In: J. E. Johnson, S. G. Eberle, T. S. Henricks, & D. Kuschne (Eds.), *The Handbook of the Study of Play* (pp. 101-120). Lanham, MD: Rowman & Littlefield Publishing Group.

Hirsh-Pasek, K., Golinkoff, R. M., Berk, L. E., & Singer, D.G. (2009). *A mandate for playful learning in preschool: Presenting the evidence*. New York, NY: Oxford University Press.

Huizinga, J. (1967). *Homo ludens*. Milano, I: Il Saggiatore (orig. ed., *Homo ludens. A study of the play elements in culture*, 1939).

Kane, P. (2004). *The Play Ethic: A Manifesto For a Different Way of Living*. London, UK: Macmillan.

Karmiloff-Smith, A. (1992). *Beyond modularity: A developmental perspective on cognitive science.* Cambridge, MA: MIT Press.
Kuschner, D. (2015). Play and Early Childhood Education. In: J. E. Johnson, S. G., Eberle, T. S., Henricks, & D., Kuschne (Eds.), *The Handbook of the Study of Play* (pp. 287-298). Lanham, MD: Rowman & Littlefield Publishing Group.
Levy, J. (1978). *Play Behavior*. New York, NY: Wiley.
Lillard, A. S. (2001). Pretend play and theory of mind: Explaining the connection. In: S. Reifel (Ed.), *Play and culture studies. Vol. 3* (pp. 350-371). Westport, CT: Ablex.
Lillemyr, O. F. (2009). *Taking Play Seriously: Children and Play in Early Childhood Education - An Exciting Challenge*. Charlotte, NC: Information Age Publishing.
Marshall, P. (2009). *Positive psychology and constructivist developmental psychology: A theoretical enquiry into how a developmental stage conception might provide further insights into specific areas of positive psychology.* Retrieved from: https://dts.lectica.org/PDF/DissertationPaul-Marshall.pdf.
Meakins, C. R. H., Bundy, A. C., & Gliner, J. (2005). Validity and Reliability of the Experience of Leisure Scale (TELS). In: F.F. McMahon, D.E. Lytle, B. Sutton-Smith, B. (Eds.), *Play. An Interdisciplinary Synthesis. Play and Culture Studies* (Vol. 6, pp. 255-267). Lanham, MD: University Press of America.
Metra, M. (2006). *Approches théoriques du jeu*. Retrieved from:
www2.ac-lyon.fr/etab/ien/ain/bourg2/IMG/pdf/Approches_theoriques_du_jeu.pdf.
Miller, E., & Almon, J. (2009). *Crisis in kindergarten: Why children need to play in school.* College Park, MD: Alliance for Childhood.
Miller, S. (1973). Ends, Means, and Galumphing: Some Leitmotifs of Play. *American Anthropologist*, 75, 87-98.
Milner, M. (1952). Aspects of Symbolism in Comprehension of the Not-self. *International Journal of Psycho-Analysis*, 33(2), 181-195.
Montessori, M. (1998). *The Secret of Childhood*. Orient Longman: Himayatnagar (or. ed., 1936).
Montessori, M. (1967). *The Absorbent Mind*. New York, NY: Dell (or. ed., 1949).
O'Connel, B., & Bretherton, I. (1984). Toddler's play, alone and with mother: The role of maternal guidance. In: I. Bretherton (Ed.), *Symbolic play: The development of social understanding* (pp. 337-369). Orlando, FL: Academic Press.
OECD (Organisation for Economic Co-operation and Development) (2010). *Recognising Non-Formal and Informal Learning: Outcomes, Policies and Practices*. Paris, F: OECD.
Parten, M. B. (1932). Social participation among pre-school children. *Journal of Abnormal and Social Psychology*, 27, 243-269.
Pellegrini, A. D. (2009). Research and policy on children's play. *Child Development Perspectives*, 3(2), 131-136.
Perroni, E. (2014). *Play: Psychoanalytic Perspectives, Survival and Human Development*. New York, NY: Routledge.
Petrie, P. (1987). *Baby play-activities for discovery and development during the first year life.* London, UK: Fances Lincon.
Piaget, J. (1972). *La formation du symbole chez l'enfant. Imitation, jeu, rêve, image et représentation.* Neûchatel, CH: Delachaux et Niestlé (or. ed., 1945).
Piaget, J. (1962). *Play, dreams and imitation in childhood*, New York, NY: Norton.
Piaget, J. (1976). *Symbolic Play*. In: J.S. Bruner, A. Jolly, & K. Silva (Eds.), *Play. Its role in Development and Evolution* (pp. 555-569). New York, NY: Basic Books.
Pope Edwards, C. (2002). Three Approaches from Europe: Waldorf, Montessori, and Reggio Emilia. *Early Childhood Research and Practice*, 4, 1.
Provenzo, E. F. (2009). Friedrich Froebel's Gifts. Connecting the Spiritual and Aesthetic to the Real World of Play and Learning. *American Journal of Play*, Summer, 85-99.

Pullen, P. S., Justice, L. M. (2003). Enhancing phonological awareness, print awareness, and oral language skills in preschool children. *Intervention in School and Clinic*, 39(2), 87-98.
Rogers, S., & Evans, J. (2007). Rethinking role play in the reception class. *Educational Research*, 49(2), 153–167.
Rubin, K. H., Fein, G. G., & Vandenberg, B. (1983). Play. In: E.M. Hetherington (Ed.), *Handbook of child psychology. Vol. 4. Socialization, personality, and social development* (pp. 693-774). New York, NY: Wiley.
Ryall, E., Russell, W., & MacLean, M. (2013). *The Philosophy of Play*. London, UK & New York, NY: Routledge.
Saracho, O. N., & Spodek, B. (2006). Young children's literacy-related play. *Early Child Development and Care*, 176(7), 707-721.
Schaffer, H. R. (1977). *Studies in mother-infant interaction*. London, UK: Academic Press.
Sluss, D. J. (2005). *Supporting Play: Birth to Age Eight.* Clifton Park, NY: Delmar Cengage Learning.
Smilansky, S. (1968). *The effects of sociodramatic play on disadvantaged Preschool children*. New York, NY: Wiley.
Smirnova, E. O, & Gudareva, O. V. (2004). Igra i proizvol'nost u sovremennykh doshkol'nikov [Play and intentionality in modern preschoolers]. *Voprosy Psychologii*, 1, 91-103.
Snow, K. (2011). *Making Play Work. What the Research Says (and does not say).* Communication presented at the 2011 NAEYC Annual Conference & Expo. Retrieved from: www.naeyc.org/content/research-news-you-can-use-play-vs-learning.
Spitz, R. A. (1945). Hospitalism—An Inquiry Into the Genesis of Psychiatric Conditions in Early Childhood. *Psychoanalytic Study of the Child*, 1, 53-74.
Staccioli, G. (2004). *Il gioco e il giocare. Elementi di didattica ludica* [Play and playing. Elements of play didactics]. Roma, I: Carocci.
Suits, B. (1977). Appendix I: Words on Play. *Journal of the Philosophy of Sport*, 4, 117-131.
Sullivan, H. S. (1953). *The interpersonal theory of psychiatry*. New York, NY: Norton.
Sutton-Smith, B. (1979). *Play and learning: The Johnson and Johnson Pediatric Round Table III*. New York, NY: Gardner.
Sutton-Smith, B. (1997). *The Ambiguity of Play*. Cambridge and London, UK: Harvard University Press.
Sutton-Smith, B. (1999). Evolving a consilience of play definitions: Playfully. *Play and Culture Studies*, 2, 239-256.
Sutton-Smith, B. (2008). Play Theory: A Personal Journey and New Thoughts. *American Journal of Play*, Summer, 80-123.
Sutton-Smith, B. (2015). Play Theory: A Personal Journey and New Thoughts. In: J. E. Johnson, S. G., Eberle, T. S., Henricks, & D., Kuschne (Eds.), *The Handbook of the Study of Play* (pp. 239-270). Lanham, MD: Rowman & Littlefield Publishing Group.
Sylva, K., Tagart, B., Melhuish E., Sammons P., & Siraj-Blatchford, I. (2007). Changing models of research to inform educational policy. *Research Papers in Education*, 22(2), 155-168.
Uren, N., & Stagnitti, K. (2009). Pretend play, social competence and involvement in children aged 5-7 years: The concurrent validity of the Child-Initiated Pretend Play Assessment. *Australian Occupational Therapy Journal*, 56(1), 33-40.
Van Oers, B., & Wardekker, W. (1999). On becoming an authentic learner: semiotic activity in the early grades. *Journal of curriculum studies*, 31(2), 229-249.
Visalberghi, A. (1958). *Esperienza e valutazione* [Experience and evaluation]. Torino, I: Taylor.
Vygotskij, L. S. (2004). Imagination and creativity in childhood. *Journal of Russian and East European Psychology*, 42(1), 7-97 (or. ed,., 1930).
Vygotskij, L. S. (1967). Play and its role in the mental development of the child. *Soviet Psychology*, 5(3), 6-18 (or. ed., 1966).

Vygotskij, L. S. (1976). Play and its Role in the Mental Development of the Child. In: J.S. Bruner, A. Jolly, & K. Silva (Eds.), *Play. Its role in Development and Evolution* (pp. 537-554). New York, NY: Basic Books.

Vygotskij, L. S. (1978). *Mind in Society: The Development of Higher Psychological Processes.* Cambridge, MA: Harvard University Press.

Vygotskij, L. S. (1997). Prehistory of the Development of Written Language. In: R. W. Rieber (Ed). *The History of the Development of Higher Mental Functions. The Collected Works of L.S. Vygotskij* (Vol. 4, 131–48). Berlin, D: Springer.

White, R. W. (1959). Motivation reconsidered. The concept of competence. *Psychological Review*, 66, 297-333.

Winnicott, D. W. (1971). *Playing and Reality.* London, UK: Tavistock Publications.

Wood, E. (2008). *The Routledge Reader in Early Childhood Education.* New York, NY: Routledge.

Wood, E. (2009). Developing a Pedagogy of Play. In: A. Anning, J. Cullen, & M. Fleer. (Eds). *Early Childhood Education: Society and Culture* (27-38). London, UK: Sage Publications.

Wood, E., & Attfield, J. (2005). *Play, Learning and the Early Childhood Curriculum.* London, UK: Paul Chapman Publishing.

Zigler, E., & Bishop-Josef, S. (2004). Play under siege. A historical overview. In: E. Zigler, D. Singer, & S. Bishop-Josef (Eds.), *Children's play: The roots of reading.* Washington, D.C.: Zero to Three Press.

Keith Towler

2 Children's Right to Play, Whoever They Are, Wherever They Are. The Play Rights of Children and Young People with Disabilities

This chapter outlines the importance of the United Nations Convention on the Rights of the Child (UNCRC), and in particular, Article 31 and General Comment No. 17, when we consider the play rights of children and young people with disabilities. First, the International Play Association (IPA) was delighted and honoured to be asked to present at the LUDI Conference on this important topic. The IPA is an international non-governmental organisation founded in 1961, which now has members in more than 50 countries worldwide. IPA's purpose is to protect, preserve, and promote child's right to play as a fundamental human right.[1]

It is, perhaps, worth outlining upfront what Article 31 of the UNCRC says: "That every child has the right to rest and leisure, to engage in play and recreational activities appropriate to the age of the child and to participate freely in cultural life and the arts. That member governments shall respect and promote the right of the child to participate fully in cultural and artistic life and shall encourage the provision of appropriate and equal opportunities for cultural, artistic, recreational and leisure activity".

So, it is worth stating that the UNCRC applies to all children across the world; all children, whoever they are and wherever they are, have the right to play. This right applies equally to children with disabilities. Why then, given that very clear commitment, do so many children with disabilities find that right is denied? This chapter aims to outline how the barriers to play impact on children with disabilities and puts forward the case for change as supported by the UN General Comment on Article 31.[2]

2.1 The UNCRC

UNICEF[3] reminds us that: "25 years ago, the world made a promise to children: that we would do everything in our power to protect and promote their rights to survive and thrive, to learn and grow, to make their voices heard and to reach their full potential.

1 For International Play Association (IPA) information and resources, please visit http://www.ipa-world.com.

2 Committee on the Rights of the Child (2013) General Comment No.17 (2013) on the right of the child to rest, leisure, play, recreational activities, cultural life and the arts (Art. 31).

3 www.unicef.org.

In spite of the overall gains, there are many children who have fallen even further behind. Old challenges have combined with new problems to deprive many children of their rights and the benefits of development".

The UNCRC outlines all the human, social, and economic rights of all children (under 18) throughout the world. It was created in 1989, and nations across all UN member states except for the United States have ratified the Convention (Somalia is in the process of finalising ratification of the Convention). There are 54 'articles' or rights in the Convention. Articles 1–42 outline the rights specific to children, and Articles 43–54 outline the obligations of State Parties and other 'duty bearers'.

2.2 Barriers, Voice, and Play Practice

The UNCRC:
- informs and guides our professional practice, values, experience, and reflections
- provides all practitioners, leaders, and services with a common platform to working with, and for, children and young people (Hanson, 2014)
- enables us to place children and young people at the heart of everything we do (Trodd & Chivers, 2011)
- enables us to navigate professional complexities and to work towards securing what is in the best interests of children and young people – to do the right thing

Until recently (2008–February 2015), I was the Children's Commissioner for Wales, and in that role, I became acutely aware of how important play is to children. In fact, there were two main things that children of primary school age wanted to talk to me about. The first is how important it is to feel safe, and the second is play. Very often, these two things go hand in hand. Feeling safe in school and learning through play is one example, and playing outdoors, maybe on our streets, without being worried about by disapproving adults is another.

There are a number of specific barriers that impact negatively on the ability of children with disabilities to enjoy their right to play. They include (and this is not an exhaustive list) physical barriers that prevent children using wheelchairs or walking aids from accessing play spaces; poor public transport (a particular issue in rural and semi-rural locations); poverty impacting on the ability to pay for and access some organised play and recreation opportunities; isolation within the family and within the community; and poor or limited assistive technologies, which reduce opportunities for participation by children with disabilities. One of the major barriers that exists is the attitude of professionals and others within the community towards disability. Negative stereotypes hurt and impact on children's lives, reduce opportunities to participate, and increase emotional stress and poor mental health.

We know that play is fundamental (not optional) to children's physical, social, mental, and emotional development. Of course, play can and should happen all the time, and children's innate desire to play must be encouraged and allowed to develop at the child's direction. We also know that this extends to all children, regardless of ability, and so, children with disabilities have an absolute right to enjoy their Article 31 rights.

An area that sometimes causes confusion is where rehabilitation and therapy for children with disabilities fits with their right to play. Some of those therapeutic and rehabilitative programmes can and do have playful qualities within them. It is important to recognise, however, that these must never be seen as a substitute for play, as described in the General Comment.

Article 12 of the UNCRC also reminds us that all children have the right to have their voice heard in any matter that affects their lives. Voice is important, and in our play practice, we must place listening and acting on the concerns and issues that children raise as central to our work with, and for, them. Children with disabilities can and do share their experiences, hopes, feelings, and wishes.

- "I love it when it snows", child aged 6.
- "...no way for me to join in", child aged 9.
- "I can never go on my own... but sometimes they can't take me and I feel sad", boy aged 15.
- "It can be scary to play outside", girl aged 8.
- "People have spit at me. I don't like that", boy aged 9.
- "I love playing with my mum", girl aged 10.
- "Playing is so good, we need more time to play, playing anywhere is just brilliant", boy aged 9.
- "Computers are good but outdoors is the best", girl aged 12.
- "I'm so happy when I'm playing. It makes me feel like sunshine inside", boy aged 6.

All of these quotes come from my meetings with children with disabilities in Wales. They are so powerful and illustrate why we must develop our play practice to meet the concerns they outline. Perhaps, we should all work to make sure that every child with a disability feels like they have sunshine within them.

2.3 Article 31 and General Comment No. 17

The UN Committee on the Rights of the Child is concerned about the poor recognition given by governments to Article 31 rights. Rising urban populations, violence in all its forms, the commercialisation of play provision, child labour, and increasing educational demands are all affecting children's opportunities to enjoy their Article 31 rights. In general, where investment is made, it is in the provision of structured and organised activities, but equally important is the need to create time and space for children to engage in spontaneous play, recreation, and creativity, and to promote societal attitudes that support and encourage such activity.

To address these concerns, the Committee produced a General Comment, which it adopted at its 62nd session (14 January–1 February 2013). The General Comment has three core objectives:

1. To enhance understanding of the importance of Article 31 for children's wellbeing and development
2. To ensure respect for and strengthen the application of the rights under Article 31, as well as other rights in the Convention
3. To highlight the implications for the determination of obligations of governments, the roles and responsibilities of the private sector, and guidelines for all individuals working with children

Within the General Comment, the Committee outlines those children who require particular attention to realise their Article 31 rights. They include girls, children living in poverty, children from indigenous and minority communities, children in situations of conflict, humanitarian and natural disasters, children in institutions, and children with disabilities.

With regard to children with disabilities, the General Comment refers to multiple barriers, including those I highlighted earlier. They point out that children with disabilities may find themselves excluded from school, and informal and social arenas where friendships are formed and where play and recreation take place. While adults sometimes overlook its importance, the opportunity to make friends and simply play together with peers is crucial to our experience of childhood and a sense of being fully part of society. Article 23 of the Convention highlights disabled children's rights to fullest participation in the community, and IPA believes that the right to play is fundamental to realisation of that right.

The General Comment highlights the problems of isolation at home, cultural attitudes, and negative stereotypes, which are hostile to and rejecting of children with disabilities; and physical inaccessibility of many environments. Lack of assistive technologies can also impede children with disabilities access to media.

Of course, many children with disabilities live in institutions, and the General Comment says that children living in residential homes and schools, hospitals, detention centres, remand homes, and refugee centres often have limited, or are denied, opportunities for play, recreation, and participation in cultural and artistic life.

The General Comment also outlines government obligations. These include governments adopting specific measures aimed at respecting and realising every child's Article 31 rights, including support for caregivers and awareness raising to challenge widespread poor cultural attitudes. Governments are also required to protect and fulfil Article 31 rights through, for example, legislation, regulation, child protection measures, professional codes, independent complaints mechanisms, data collection, and appropriate budget and resource allocations. It points out the importance of Universal Design to promote and protect children's play, municipal planning, improvement of school and community environments, and training and capacity building for all professionals working with or for children, or whose work impacts on children.

2.4 Conclusion

We need to build a worldwide campaign on Article 31. The publication of the General Comment provides an ideal opportunity to further raise awareness of the importance of Article 31 with state parties, government departments, civil society, and the general public across the world.

The case to make sure that children with disabilities have a right to play is surely beyond question. The link with their health, wellbeing, and development makes children's play fundamental, not optional. The responsibility to ensure this happens rests with family members, caregivers, professionals, policy makers, and governments.

If we managed to implement the vision set in the General Comment on Article 31, we would have happy children, learning through play and realising their individual potential whoever they are and wherever they live.

References

Hanson, K. (2014). 'Killed by Charity'. Towards Interdisciplinary children's rights studies. *Childhood*, 21(4), 441-446.

Trodd, L., & Chivers, L. (2011). *Interprofessional Working in Practice. Learning and working together for children and families*. New York, NY: Mc Graw Hill, Open University Press.

Daniela Bulgarelli and Nicole Bianquin

3 Conceptual Review of Play

3.1 Definition of Play

LUDI adopted the definition of play proposed by Garvey (1990), as it has been considered the most representative one for the purposes of the project: "Play is a range of voluntary, intrinsically motivated activities normally associated with recreational pleasure and enjoyment". This definition shows interesting features: it can include all kinds of activities performed with ludic intention and takes into consideration three important and typical dimensions of the infant play: pleasure, self-direction, and intrinsic drive. On the contrary, all the activities made in ludic contexts and/or in a ludic mood, with ludic tools (toys, games, etc.), but driven by an extrinsic goal (i.e., educational, rehabilitative) are defined as 'play-like' activities, and are not the core of the LUDI research activity.

The International Classification of Functioning, Disability and Health – Children and Youth Version (ICF-CY, WHO, 2007) includes play – that is not considered in the version for adult – thus underlying the great importance it has in childhood. Defined as a component of the domain 'Activities and Participation', play is placed both in Chapter 1 'Learning and applying knowledge' and in Chapter 8 'Major life areas'. In the first case, play is seen as an engine for the child's development, in particular, for learning: in the item 'Learning through actions with objects' (d131), the ICF-CY includes learning through actions with single, two or more objects, and also through symbolic play (actions relating objects, toys, or materials symbolically) as well as pretend play (actions involving pretence, substituting an object, body part, or body movement to enact a situation or event). In the second case, play is interpreted as 'Engagement in play' (d880), that is "Purposeful, sustained engagement in activities with objects, toys, materials or games, occupying oneself or with other" (2007:184). This second definition is more adherent to the aims of our project and is then inserted as a further definition of play adopted by LUDI. The item 'Engagement in play' is subdivided into: play (d8800), onlooker play (d8801), parallel play (d8802), shared cooperative play (8803); these categories will be better illustrated in the following paragraph. In relation to the objectives of LUDI, it is worth mentioning the fact that play is also treated within the domain of Environmental Factors in Chapter 1, 'Product and technology': in fact, this chapter considers the following items: 'Equipment, products and technologies used in structured or unstructured play by an individual or group' (2007:192) and 'Products and technology used for play' (d1152). Both adapted and non-adapted toys, or specially designed technologies to assist play can be described.

3.2 Classifications of Types of Play

The definition of play that LUDI adopted underlined the fundamental characteristics that were reported in Chapter 1. Taking those key characteristics for granted to define an activity as 'play', children's play could be performed and described at different levels of cognitive complexity or of social engagement, independently from some kinds of impairment.

Both pedagogy and psychology have a long tradition in the study of play, and have developed many classifications of play, that can be clustered around two main dimensions: the first concerns the cognitive complexity implied by the different types of play and the second concerns the degree and type of social interaction in which the child is involved while playing. In some cases, these classifications described the different types also as developmental stages, and related them to the general cognitive and/or social child development; in other cases, these types could be considered as coexisting and overlapping, at least partially.

Piaget's original cognitive classification of play was organised in stages characterised by growing complexity, and it has been partly changed by other scholars who developed substages – or subtypes – to better catch different qualities of play, or inserted new stages or types to include the interactional dimension (Rubin et al., 1976; Santrock, 2006; Smilansky, 1945; Stagnitti & Unsworth, 2000, 2009; Takata, 1974). The social classification of play has been originally proposed by Parten in the early 1930s, and it still remains the main reference in this area of studies. This classification was organised in stages of growing complexity as well. Garvey's proposal differed from the others, as the author did not adopt the dimensions, cognitive or social, but chose to single out and describe broad types of play behaviours; furthermore, they were not hierarchically organised. A further group of classifications of play strictly relates to the type of toys used while playing (ESAR System, 2002; Kudrowitz & Wallace, 2009; U.S. Consumer Product Safety Commission). Table 3.1 summarises the types of play described in the considered classifications, the principal developmental dimension that describes them, and whether they are hierarchically organised.

In what follows, some more information about the definitions of the types of play according to the various authors are reported.

a. Piaget (1945) – the following categories are hierarchically ordered:
- Practice play: listening, visual, and tactile experimentation of objects, sounds, words, expressions.
- Symbolic play: pretend play; make-believe activities (symbolic use of objects as they were something else); use of absent objects.
  - Play with rules: games with a specific code and rules accepted and followed by the players.

Table 3.1. Classification of types of play

	Author(s)	Year	Dimension	Stages	Types
a	Piaget	1945	Cognitive	Yes	Practice play; Symbolic play; Play with rules
b	Smilansky	1968	Cognitive	Yes	Functional play; Constructive play; Symbolic play; Games with rules
c	Takata	1974	Cognitive	Yes	Sensorimotor play; Symbolic and simple constructive play; Dramatic and complex constructive play; Games with rules; Recreational and competitive play
d	Rubin et al.	1976 1983	Cognitive	Yes	Sensorimotor play; Simulation; Simulation with objects; Simulation with substitution; Sociodramatic; Role-playing; Games with rules
e	Garvey	1990	Behavioural	No	Play with motion and interaction; Play with objects; Play with language; Play with social materials
f	Santrock	2006	Cognitive and social	Yes	Sensorimotor play; Pretend/Symbolic play; Social play; Constructive play
g	Stagnitti & Unsworth	2000 2009	Cognitive (only pretend play)	Yes	Symbolic play; Sociodramatic play; Role play; Fantastic play
h	Garon et al. (ESAR)	1982 2002	Cognitive	Yes	Exercise play; Symbolic play; Assembly (=construction); Games with rules
i	U.S. National Institute of Play	N.A.	Cognitive and social	Yes	Attunement play; Body play; Object play; Social play; Imaginative and pretend play; Storytelling play; Creative play
j	Parten & Mildred	1932	Social	Yes	Solitary play; Parallel play; Associative play; Cooperative play
k	ICF-CY	2007	Social	N.A.	Solitary play; Onlooker play; Parallel play; Shared cooperative play
l	Smith	2002	Cognitive	Yes, within each stage	Early exploratory/Practice Play; Construction Play; Pretend & Role Play; Game & Activity Play; Sport & Recreational Play; Media Play; Educational & Academic Play
m	Kudrowitz & Wallace	2009	Toys	N.A.	Construction; Fantasy; Sensory; Challenge
n	Goodson & Bronson	1997	Toys	N.A.	Active Play; Manipulative Play; Make-believe Play; Creative Play; Learning Play

b. Smilansky (1968) developed Piaget's categories and splitted the first play stage into two ones.
- Functional play: simple body movements or actions with objects.
- Constructive play: doing something with objects (i.e., building a tower of small cubes).
- Symbolic play (Piaget's examples).

c. Games with rules (Piaget's examples). Takata (1974), based on a review of literature, proposed an age-based classification of play:
- Sensorimotor play (0-2 years).
- Symbolic and simple constructive play (2-4 years).
- Dramatic and complex constructive play (4-7 years).
- Games with rules (7-12 years).
- Recreational and competitive play (12-16 years).

d. Rubin et al. (1976, 1983) developed Piaget's symbolic stage into five stages with growing complexity:
- Sensorimotor play: it is similar to Piaget's practice play.
- Simulation of actions by the child; in this stage, only the body is involved.
- Simulation with objects (with dolls or other toys).
- Simulation with substitution, in which the objects become other than what they are.
- Sociodramatic play, where children act out roles in life scenes.
- Role-playing, in which the child takes the next step of assigning roles to others and planning scenes.
- Games with rules (Piaget's definition).

e. Garvey's proposal (1990) describes broad types of play behaviours:
- Play with motion and interaction: it reflects exuberance; running, jumping, skipping, shrieking, and laughing are expressions of this type of play.
- Play with objects: children can explore objects with their senses, can manipulate them, practice and use the objects as they are meant to, and repeat these behaviours several times.
- Play with language can be expressed in four different forms: play with sounds and noises; play with linguistic systems, such as those involving word meanings or grammatical constructions; play with rhymes and words; play with the conventions of speech.
- Play with social materials: this type of play is centred on the social world and consists in make-believe and pretending.

f. Santrock (2006) reclaimed Piaget's classification and added social and constructive play:
- Sensorimotor play: exploratory and playful visual and motor transactions; exploration of objects and their functioning; exploring causes and effects.

- Pretend/symbolic play: transforming objects, substituting them for other objects, and acting towards them as if they were these other objects.
- Social play: play that involves interactions with peers.
- Constructive play: combines sensorimotor/practice repetitive play with symbolic representation of ideas: children engage in self-regulated creation or construction of a product or a problem solution.

g. Stagnitti and Unsworth (2000, 2009) proposed four types of play:
- Symbolic play: children playing 'as if' and using an imaginary approach to play.
- Sociodramatic play.
- Role play.
- Fantastic play.

h. The ESAR system has been proposed by Garon et al. (2002) and is at the basis of the 'Guide to Play and Toys' developed by the Instituto Tecnològico del Juguete (AIJU) developed in Spain to classify toys; the acronym is related to the four categories of play identified by Smilansky:
- Exercise play: sensory and motor exercise play.
- Symbolic play: play that allows imitating objects, persons, or roles, which allows creating scenarios and representing reality through images or symbols.
- Assembly (= construction): play to gather, combine, arrange, and fit more elements to form a whole, and achieve a specific goal.
- Games with rules (Piaget's definition).

i. The U.S. National Institute of Play classified patterns of play:
- Attunment play: joint attention interactions between infant and mother.
- Body play: exploratory body movements, rhythmic early speech (moving vocal cords), locomotor, and rotational activity.
- Object play: activities involving objects.
- Social play: activities carried out with parents, pets, peers.
- Imaginative and pretend play: make-believe activities.
- Storytelling play: activities related to listening and telling stories.
- Creative play: activities that give the possibility to access fantasy-play, to transcend the reality of our ordinary lives, and in the process, germinate new ideas and shape and re-shape them.

j. Parten (1932) was the first scholar to consider and describe different types of the infant play under its social aspect:
- Solitary play: the child plays alone and independently even if surrounded by other children.
- Parallel play: the child plays independently at the same activity, at the same time, and at the same place.

- Associative play: the child is still focused on a separate activity, but there is a considerable amount of sharing, lending, taking turns, and attending to the activities of one's peers.
- Cooperative play: children can organise their play and/or activity cooperatively with a common goal and are able differentiate and assign roles.

k. The International Classification of Functioning, Disability and Health Children and Youth Version (2007) describes four categories of play in Activities and Participation in the item of Engagement of play (d880):
- Solitary play: occupying oneself in purposeful, sustained engagement in activities with objects, toys, materials, or games.
- Onlooker play: occupying oneself by purposeful observation of the activities of others with objects, toys, materials, or games, but not joining in their activities.
- Parallel play: engaging in purposeful, sustained activities with objects, toys, materials, or games in the presence of other persons also engaged in play, but not joining in their activities.
- Shared cooperative play: joining others in sustained engagement in activities with objects, toys, materials, or games with a shared goal or purpose.

l. Smith (2002) produced a study for the U.S. Consumer Product Safety Commission in which the following play stages are described:
- Early exploratory/practice play: includes all the first stages of the child's manipulative and exploratory play, such as mirrors, mobiles, pull and push toys.
- Construction play: play activities with blocks and interlocking building materials.
- Pretend and role play: all the activities that imply symbolic and/or narrative competence, such as dolls and stuffed toys, play scenes and puppets, dress-up materials, small vehicles, and so on.
- Game and activity play: toys belonging to this type can be puzzles, card, floor, board, and table games; computer and video games.
- Sport and recreational play: ride-on toys, recreational and sport equipment belong to this type of play.
- Media play: in this category, Smith includes arts and crafts, audio-visual equipment, musical instruments.
- Educational and academic play: books, learning toys, smart toys, and educational software.

As underlined before, there are also classifications based on toys. In many cases, these classifications do not belong to a scientific framework and have been developed through a bottom-up strategy, that is, by considering mainly the characteristics of use suggested by the toys themselves. Consequently, generally speaking, such classifications are difficult to compare with others. Furthermore, as different toys can be suggested for different age ranges, it is also difficult to identify whether these classifications refer to stages or not.

m. Kudrowitz and Wallace (2009) proposed four features to describe the values of play and/or toys:
- Construction: this play is about creating and not simply creativity.
- Fantasy: this play is about role-playing or it has a level of pretence.
- Sensory: this play involves aesthetics and entertaining the senses.
- Challenge: this can be physical or mental; physical challenges include both fine and gross motor skill development.

n. Goodson and Bronson – U.S. Consumer Product Safety Commission – proposed another classification of toys (1997) from which Smith's work was then developed:
- Active play: push and pull, ride-on toys; outdoor and gym, sports equipment.
- Manipulative play: construction toys, pattern making, dressing, lacing, stringing, sand and water play toys.
- Make-believe play: dolls, puppets, stuffed toys, place scenes, transportation toys.
- Creative play: musical instruments, art and craft materials, audio-visual equipment.
- Learning play: games, books, specific skill-development toys.

3.3 LUDI Classification of Types of Play

LUDI aims at proposing a classification of types of play to create a common language among practitioners and scholars, who daily work in the field of play of children with disabilities. A shared and nuanced understanding of play is important to better support the right to play. In fact, reasoning in terms of typologies of play could be crucial for several purposes: for instance, to better understand how to support, for the sake of play, a specific kind of play of children with their specific characteristics and abilities; or to design accessible toys that can allow activities at different play levels according to the children's abilities. This will also be the classification used in the following chapters.

Starting from the analysis of the existing classifications, their contents and different types of play they include and describe, a new classification has been developed for LUDI according to two main scopes:

- It should be exhaustive; thus, including most of the types of play identified by scholars over the years.
- It should be consistent and effective, for the purposes of the project.

Furthermore, the LUDI Classification should maintain the two main clusters around which the types of play have been grouped, corresponding to the main dimensions the researchers decided to underline. The LUDI Classification – as it is possible to see in Table 3.2 – is strongly inspired for the cognitive dimension by the Piaget/Smilansky classifications, and for the social dimension by that of Parten.

Table 3.2. LUDI Classification of play

Dimension	Type of play
Cognitive	Practice Symbolic Constructive Play with rules (including video games)
Social	Solitary Parallel Associative Cooperative

Anyway, in the LUDI Classification, each type of play should be considered as a more comprehensive category than the types of play reported in the literature: in fact, each LUDI type of play includes types and definitions that other researchers have singled out. In Table 3.3, a first attempt is made to group these types around the LUDI types.

Table 3.3. Play theoretical references

Cognitive dimension	
Practice	Practice play (Piaget); Functional play (Smilansky); Sensorimotor play (Takata; Rubin et al.; Santrock); Play with motion and interaction, Play with objects (Garvey); Attunement play, Body play, Object play (U.S. Institute of Play); Exercise play (ESAR); Early exploratory/Practice Play (Smith)
Symbolic	Symbolic play (Piaget, Smilansky); Symbolic and simple constructive play, Dramatic and complex constructive play (Takata); Simulation, Simulation with objects, Simulation with substitution, Sociodramatic, Role-playing (Rubin et al.); Play with language, Play with social materials (Garvey); Pretend/ symbolic play (Santrock); Symbolic play, Sociodramatic play, Role play, Fantastic play (Stagnitti); Symbolic play, Imaginative and pretend play (U.S. Institute of Play); Symbolic play (ESAR); Pretend and Role Play (Smith)
Constructive	Constructive play (Smilansky, Santrock); Symbolic and simple constructive play, Dramatic and complex constructive play (Takata); Object play (U.S. Institute of Play); Assembly play (ESAR); Construction play (Smith)
Games with rules	Play with rules (Piaget); Games with rules (Smilansky; Takata; Rubin et al.; ESAR); Game and Activity play (Smith)

The description of each type of play adopted in the LUDI Classification, for what concerns the cognitive dimension, has been built upon the definition from the literature reported earlier, and is better described in what follows.

a. Practice play – cognitive dimension

This type of play refers to two main aspects:

- simple body actions or experimentation of body (movements with hands, arms, legs, head and face, vocalisations, etc.);
- visual and tactile experimentation of objects (children can explore objects with their senses, can manipulate them, practice and use the objects as they are meant to). Moreover, children explore causes and effects (i.e., drop an object and listen to the sound it produces).

Typically, in this type of play, movements and experimentations are repeated several times. This type of play is typical in the first and second year of life.

b. Symbolic play – cognitive dimension

This type of play implies giving new signification to objects, persons, actions, or events: thus, children symbolically use objects as they were something else, produce pretend play, and make-believe activities.

There are several levels of symbolic play with growing complexity:

- simulation of actions by the child; in this stage, only the body is involved
- simulation with objects
- simulation with substitution, in which the objects become other than what they are
- use of absent objects

Role-playing or sociodramatic play is another type of symbolic play, where children act out roles in life scenes; they assign roles to others and plan scenes. It involves narrative competence.

The more simple expressions of this type of play typically emerge at the end of the second year of life.

c. Constructive play – cognitive dimension

This play consists in gathering, combining, arranging, and fitting more elements to form a whole, and achieve a specific goal. It usually involves blocks and interlocking building materials (i.e., building a tower of small cubes). In this type of play, the child combines sensorimotor/practice repetitive play with symbolic representation of ideas: children engage in self-regulated creation or construction of a product or a problem solution.

d. Rule play – cognitive dimension

This play consists of games with a specific code and rules accepted and followed by the players. This type of play is usually combined with the other three types: practice, symbolic, and constructive.

The four types of cognitive play emerged in specific period of the life of the typically developing children, as the cognitive abilities develop and become stable: practice play appears since the first weeks, because it basically involves sensory and motor competence and requires less complex cognitive abilities. Usually, symbolic play appears between 18 and 24 months, as the child's representative ability emerges. Constructive play appears in the second year as well, whereas first types of rule play emerge in the preschool age, from three years, when the child is able to manage easy rules.

Each type of cognitive play appears in a simplest 'version' during the childhood and develops and becomes more and more complex throughout lifetime. Early examples of symbolic play usually involve the child pretending to do something related to everyday routines: cooking and eating fake food, pretending to go sleeping, etc. During infancy, symbolic play becomes more and more complex: children engage in role-playing with peers, building very complex fantastic scenarios, with rules to be followed by all the participants (e.g., pretending to be at school with teachers and pupils or pretending to be fairies and wizards in a magical world).

The few examples reported here show that each kind of cognitive play is rarely played independently, but very often intertwines with other types of play. Thus, the symbolic play of pretending to be mom and dad with their kinds involves aspects of rule play because each child will follow the social rules related to his or her character (mom and dad will take care of the children and the house; the children will play and disobey to some rules, etc.); aspects of constructive play (putting together different elements in play); and aspects of practice play (the kids play with the ball during the session of symbolic play).

As it has been synthesised in Table 3.2, play can be categorised accordingly to the cognitive dimension or social dimension, the description of which has been strongly influenced by Parten's studies. The description that is proposed here is also derived from the ICF-CY. In what follows, the social dimensions of play are described.

a. Solitary – social dimension

Occupying oneself in purposeful, sustained engagement in activities with objects, toys, materials, or games. The child plays alone and independently even if surrounded by other children.

b. Parallel – social dimension

Engaging in purposeful, sustained activities with objects, toys, materials, or games in the presence of other persons also engaged in play, but not joining in their activities. The child plays independently at the same activity, at the same time, and at the same place.

c. Associative – social dimension

The child is still focused on a separate activity, but there is a considerable amount of sharing, lending, taking turns, and attending to the activities of one's peers.

d. Cooperative – social dimension

Joining others in sustained engagement in activities with objects, toys, materials, or games with a shared goal or purpose. Children can organise their play and/or activity cooperatively with a common goal and are able differentiate and assign roles.

Each type of cognitive play can be played at a different social level: in solitary, parallel, associative, and cooperative way. For instance, practice play involves two persons in associative way in the case of the peek-a-boo game, or whenever children play clapping their hands together, crossing hands fast. Again, the child can play symbolically with dolls on his or her own (solitary), or he/she can play with other children, each child doing the same activities with the dolls but independently (parallel play), each child playing with his or her doll sharing the activities with the peers (associative play), or the children taking along cooperative activities with the doll (one child cleans the doll, while the other cooks some food for it).

Very often, the possibility to play with other persons allows the children to make the play more complex, from a cognitive perspective as well, because each player brings ideas and cues according to his or her ability, habits, and so on: this is the case of the child playing with peers, older children, or adults.

3.4 Type of Play: Areas of Development and Child's Abilities

Table 3.4 describes the children's area of psychological and physical development and the abilities that are necessary to display the types of play. For each play, the child needs to possess the main area of development and at least some of the abilities.

Table 3.4. Areas of development prevailingly involved by type of play

Type of play	Areas of development prevailingly involved	Abilities
Practice	Psychomotor Cognitive (in the first year of life) Cause/effect relationship Permanence of the object	Experimentation Exploration Exercise Repetition Imitation
	Sensorial	Observation Listening Touching Feeling (e.g., with mouth)
Symbolic	Symbolic/representative Pretending (understand and use pretend and make-believe) Representation Drawing (from scribble to extensive drawings) Language (from wording to discourse)	Invention Imagination Interpretation (e.g., of roles) Imitation

continued Table 3.4. Areas of development prevailingly involved by type of play

Type of play	Areas of development prevailingly involved	Abilities
Construction	Fine and complex psychomotor	Gathering Assembling Combining Arranging Fitting Stringing Plugging Sticking Use of tools (hammer, screwdriver, spanner, and so on)
	Cognitive and meta-cognitive Goal-directed Planning Problem solving Spatial cognition Self-regulation	Invention Imagination Hypothesis making Self-monitoring, self-evaluation Identification and correction of errors
Rule	Cognitive and meta-cognitive Understanding and adhesion to conventions Understanding of and adhesion to rule systems Strategic thought	Competition Collaboration Team work (participation, organisation) Risk-taking
	Social and meta-social Becoming and being part of groups and systems (game teams, and so on) Understanding and interpreting the others' role	

References

Garon, D., Chiasson, R., & Filion, R. (2002). *Le système ESAR. Guide d'analyse, de classification et d'organisation d'une collection de jeux et jouets*. Paris, F: Electre.

Garvey, C. (1990). *Play*. Cambridge, MA: Harvard University Press.

Goodson, B. & Bronson, M. (1997). *Which toy for which child*. Technical Report, 285-286, U.S. Consumer Product Safety Commission.

Kudrowitz, B. M., & Wallace, D. R. (2009). The play pyramid: A play classification and ideation tool for toy design. *International Journal of Arts and Technology*, 3(1), 36-56.

Parten, M. B. & Mildred, J. (1932). Social play among preschool children. *Journal of Abnormal and Social Psychology*, 27, 243–69.

Piaget, J. (1945). *Play, dreams and imitation in childhood*. London, UK: Taylor & Francis.

Rubin, K. H., Fein, G., & Vanderberg, B. (1983). Free play behaviours in middle and lower class pre-schoolers: Parten and Piaget revisited. *Child Development*, 47, 414-419.

Rubin, K. H., Fein, G., & Vanderberg B. (1983). Play. In: P. Mussen, & E. M. Hetherington (Eds.) *Handbook of Child Psychology*, vol. 4., Socialization, personality, and social development (pp. 693-774). New York, NY: Wiley.

Smilansky, S. (1968). *The effects of sociodramatic play on disadvantaged preschool children*. New York, NY: Wiley.

Smith, P. K., Takhvar, M., Gore, N., & Vollstedt, R. (1985). Play in young children: Problems of definition, categorisation and measurement. *Early Child Development and Care*, 19, 25-41.

Stagnitti, K., & Unsworth, C. (2004). The importance of pretend play in child development: an occupational therapy perspective. *American Journal of Occupational Therapy*, 63, 121-127.

Stagnitti, K. & Unsworth, C. (2000). The importance of pretend play in child development: An occupational therapy perspective. *British Journal of Occupational Therapy*, 63(3), 121-127.

Takata, N. (1974). Play as a prescription. In: M. Reilly (Ed.), *Play as exploratory learning* (pp. 209-246). Beverly Hills, CA: Sage Publication.

World Health Organisation (2001). *International Classification of Functioning Disability and Health*. Geneva, CH: WHO.

World Health Organisation (2007). *International Classification of Functioning Disability and Health, Children and Youth Version*. Geneva, CH: WHO.

Nicole Bianquin and Daniela Bulgarelli

4 Conceptual Review of Disabilities

4.1 LUDI Definition of Disability

LUDI chose to adopt the definition of disability proposed by the International Classification of Functioning, Disability and Health (WHO, 2001) as it fits the purposes of the project.

Two definitions of disability that the ICF offers are outlined: both emphasise the complex interconnection between the individual and the environment. The first one puts greater emphasis on the environment and on how it can constitute a barrier or a facilitator for the individual's functioning. The second one explains the ways in which disablement can manifest in relation to restrictions in participation. They are presented as follows.

a) "Disability is characterized as the outcome or the result of a complex relationship between an individual's health condition[1] and personal factors,[2] and of the external factors[3] that represent the circumstances in which the individual lives. Because of this relationship, different environments may have a very different impact on the same individual with a given health condition. An environment with barriers,[4] or without facilitators,[5] will restrict the

1 "Health condition is an umbrella term for disease (acute or chronic), disorder, injury or trauma. A health condition may also include other circumstances such as pregnancy, ageing, stress, congenital anomaly or genetic predisposition" (WHO, 2001:228).

2 "Personal factors are contextual factors that relate to the individual, such as age, gender, social, status, life experience and so on, which are not currently classified in ICF but which users may incorporate in their application of the classification" (WHO, 2001:229).

3 "Environmental factors constitute a component of ICF, and refer to all aspects of the external or extrinsic world that form the context of an individual's life and, as such, have an impact on that person's functioning. Environmental factors include the physical world and its features, the human-made physical world, other people in different relationships and roles, attitudes and values, social systems and services, and policies, rules and laws" (WHO, 2001:229).

4 "Barriers are factors in a person's environment that, through their absence or presence, limit functioning and create disability. These include aspects such as physical environment that is inaccessible, lack of relevant assistive technology, and negative attitudes of people towards disability, as well as services, systems and policies that are either nonexistent or that hinder the involvement of all people with a health condition in all areas of life" (WHO, 2001:230).

5 "Facilitators are factors in a person's environment that, through their absence or presence, improve functioning and reduce disability. These include aspects such as a physical environment that is accessible, the availability of relevant assistive technology, and positive attitudes of people towards disability, as well as services, systems and policies that aim to increase the involvement of all people with a health condition in all areas of life. Absence of a factor can also be facilitating, for example the absence of stigma or negative attitudes" (WHO, 2001:229).

individual's performance;[6] other environments that are more facilitating may increase that performance. Society may hinder an individual's performance because either it creates barriers (e.g. inaccessible buildings) or it does not provide facilitators (e.g. unavailability of assistive devices)" (WHO, 2001:15).

b) "Disability is an umbrella term for impairments,[7] activity,[8] limitations,[9] and participation[10] restrictions.[11] It denotes the negative aspects of the interaction between an individual (with a health condition) and the individual's contextual factors[12] (environmental and personal factors)" (WHO, 2001:228).

Moreover, these definitions are also evoked within the Convention on the Rights of Persons with Disabilities (UN, 2006), which puts emphasis on the possibility of participation for each individual: "[Recognizing that] disability is an evolving concept [...] [that] results from the interaction between persons with impairments and attitudinal and environmental barriers that hinders their full and effective participation in society on an equal basis with others" (Convention on the Rights of Persons with Disabilities, Preamble, Art. e).

According to the biopsychosocial model adopted by the ICF, these definitions highlight that disability is not a fixed concept. The condition of disability strictly depends on the impairment on one hand and on contextual factors on the other: the environmental characteristics (among them: social attitudes, architectural

6 "Performance is a construct that describes, as a qualifier, what individuals do in their current environment, and so brings in the aspect of a person's involvement in life situations. The current environment is also described using the Environmental Factors component" (WHO, 2001:230).

7 "Impairment is a loss or abnormality in body structure or physiological function (including mental functions). Abnormally here is used strictly to refer to a significant variation from established statistical norms (i.e. as a deviation from a population mean within measured standard norms) and should be used only in this sense" (WHO, 2001:229)

8 "Activity is the execution of a task or action by an individual. It represents the individual perspective of functioning" (WHO, 2001:229).

9 "Activity limitations are difficulties an individual may have in executing activities. An activity limitation may range from a slight to a severe deviation in terms of quality or quantity in executing the activity in a manner or to the extent that is expected of people without the health condition" (WHO, 2001:229).

10 "Participation is a person's involvement in a life situation. It represents the societal perspective of functioning" (WHO, 2001:229).

11 "Participation restrictions are problems an individual may experience in involvement in life situations. The presence of a participation restriction is determined by comparing an individual's participation to that which is expected of an individual without disability in that culture or society" (WHO, 2001:229).

12 "Contextual factors are the factors that together constitute the complete context of an individual's life, and, in particular, the background against which health states are classified in ICF. There are two components of contextual factors: Environmental Factors and Personal Factors" (WHO, 2001:229).

characteristics, social and legal structures) and the personal characteristics (among them: gender, age, coping styles, social background, education, profession, past and current experience, temperament). When this encounter between the person's functioning and the environment is not balanced, it can lead to limitation of activities and restriction in participation. This can be the case of participation in play activities of children with disabilities.

4.2 LUDI Categories of Childhood Disabilities

A classification of different types of disabilities is needed within LUDI because play, play materials, and play contexts can have a strict relationship with the individual's impairments and his or her activity possibilities.

OECD's (Organization for Economic Cooperation and Development) Centre for Educational Research and Innovation (CERI) published an interesting document 'Students with Disabilities, Learning Difficulties and Disadvantages: Policies, Statistics and Indicators' (2007, an updated version of a previous document published in 2005), which contains a collection of data from many countries. The document presents a comparison of data concerning the access to educational provisions by students with special needs in a number of OECD countries. In order for policy-relevant comparisons to emerge, a resource-based approach would require that the pupils included under this definition would need to be subdivided into some forms of straightforward classification scheme. Participating countries to the research agreed on a tri-partite system, in which students are divided into three cross-national categories: A, B, and C.

- Disabilities (category A): Pupils with disabilities or impairments that are viewed in medical terms as organic disorders attributable to organic pathologies (e.g., in relation to sensory, motor, or neurological defects)
- Difficulties (category B): Pupils with behavioural or emotional disorders, or specific difficulties in learning
- Disadvantages (category C): Pupils with disadvantages arising primarily from socio-economic, cultural, and/or linguistic factors

As LUDI focusses on the play of children with disabilities, the target audience of the project is related to category A. Table 4.1 shows the classifications used in the OECD member countries only with respect to category A.

Table 4.1. Classifications of category A used in OECD member countries

Country	Physical	Hearing	Visual	Mental	Communication	Multiple	Autism	Health	Behaviour or Emotion	Others
Austria	Physically disabled	Hearing impaired or deaf	Visually impaired or blind	Severe mental disability	- Speech impairment - Moderate speech problems			Ill students in hospital		
Belgium (Flemish community)	Pupils with a physical handicap	Auditory handicap	Visual handicap	- Minor - Moderate or serious mental handicap				Children suffering from protracted illness		
Belgium (French community)	Physical deficiencies	Hearing impairment	Visual deficiencies	- Mild - Moderate or profound mental retardation				Students suffering from an illness		
Canada (Alberta)	- Severe - Mild or moderate physical or medical disability	- Deafness - Mild or moderate hearing disability	- Blindness - Mild or moderate visual disability	- Severe - Mild - Moderate mental disability	- Severe - Mild or moderate communication disability	- Severe - Mild or moderate multiple disability				
Canada (British Columbia)	Physical disabilities or chronic health impairments	Hearing impairments	- Visual impairment - Deaf or blindness	Moderate to severe to profound intellectual disabilities		Multiple disabilities	Autism		Severe behaviour disorders	
Canada (New Brunswick)	Physical	Perceptual		Intellectual	Communicational	Multiple				

continued **Table 4.1.** Classifications of category A used in OECD member countries

Country	Physical	Hearing	Visual	Mental	Communication	Multiple	Autism	Health	Behaviour or Emotion	Others
Canada (Saskatchewan)	Orthopaedic impairments	Deaf or hard of hearing	Visual impairments	Intellectual disabilities		Multiple disabilities	Autism	Chronically ill		Traumatic brain injury
Chile	Motor deficit or disorder	Hearing deficit	Visual deficit	Mental deficiency	Serious social and communication impairments					
Czech Republic	Physical handicaps	Hearing handicaps	Sight handicaps	Mentally retarded	Speech handicaps	Multiple handicaps	Autistic	- Students in hospital - Children with poor health (pre-primary only)		Other handicaps
Finland	Physical and other impairment	Hearing impairment	Visual impairment	- Mild - Moderate or severe mental impairment	Dysphasia		Autism and Asperger's syndrome			
France	Physical handicap	- Deaf - Partially hearing	- Blind - Partially sighted	- Severe - Moderate - Mild mental handicap	Speech and language disorders	Multiply handicapped		Metabolic disorders		- Other neuro-psychological disorders - Other deficiencies
Germany	Physically handicapped	Partially hearing or deaf	Partially sighted or blind	Mentally handicapped	Handicapped in speaking	Multiple handicaps	Autism	Sick		
Greece	Physical impairments	Hearing impairments	Visual impairments	Mental impairments			Autism			Other impairments

continued **Table 4.1.** Classifications of category A used in OECD member countries

Country	Physical	Hearing	Visual	Mental	Communication	Multiple	Autism	Health	Behaviour or Emotion	Others
Hungary	Physical disability	Hearing disabilities	Visual disabilities	Moderate degree of mental disability		Multiple disabilities	Autism			
Ireland	Physically handicapped	Hearing impaired	Visually impaired	- Mild - Moderate - Severely and profoundly mentally handicapped	Specific speech and language disorder	Multiply handicapped				
Italy	- Mild - Severe physical handicap	Hearing impairment	Visual impairment	- Moderate - Severe mental handicap		Multiple handicap				
Japan	Physically disabled	Deaf and hard of hearing	Blind and partially sighted	Intellectual disabilities	Speech impaired			Health impaired	Emotionally disturbed	
Korea	Students with physical impairments	Students with hearing impairments	Students with visual impairments	Students with mental retardation	Students with speech impairments					Students with other disabilities
Luxemburg	Motor impairment	Sensory impairment		Mental impairment					Emotionally disturbed children	

continued **Table 4.1.** Classifications of category A used in OECD member countries

Country	Physical	Hearing	Visual	Mental	Communication	Multiple	Autism	Health	Behaviour or Emotion	Others
Mexico	Motor disability	- Auditory or hearing disability - Deafness or severe auditory disability	- Blindness - Partial visual disability	Intellectual disability		Multiple disability				
The Netherlands	Physically handicapped or motor impairment	- Deaf children - Hard of hearing	Visual handicap	Mental handicaps	Language and communication disabilities	Multiply handicapped		- Other health impairment - Chronic conditions requiring paediatric institutes	Behaviour disabilities	
Poland	Motion handicap	- Deaf - Partially hearing	- Blind - Partially sighted	- Light - Moderate and severe - Profound mental handicap		Multiple handicap	Autism	Chronically ill		
Slovak Republic	Physical disability	Hearing impairment	Visual impairment	- Mild - Moderate severe mental retardation	Speech disorders	Multiple impairment	Autism	Ill and physically weak children in medical facilities		

continued **Table 4.1.** Classifications of category A used in OECD member countries

Country	Physical	Hearing	Visual	Mental	Communication	Multiple	Autism	Health	Behaviour or Emotion	Others
Spain	Motor impaired	Hearing impaired	Visual impaired	Mental handicap		Multiple impairment	Serious personality disorders, psychosis, and autism	Students in hospital or with health problems		
Sweden[1]	- Pupils with impaired hearing, vision and physical disabilities - Students with impaired hearing and physical disabilities			Students with mental retardation						
Switzerland	Physical disabilities: special schools	Deaf or hard hearing: special schools	Visual handicap: special schools	-Students with a mental handicap or educable mental handicap: special schools - Students with a mental handicap or trainable mental handicap: special schools	Language disability: special schools	- Students with a mental handicap or multiply handicapped: special schools - Multiple disabilities: special schools		Chronic conditions prolonged hospitalisation: special schools	Behaviour disorders: special schools	

[1] This country is not included in the publication of 2007, but in the previous one only (2005).

continued **Table 4.1.** Classifications of category A used in OECD member countries

Country	Physical	Hearing	Visual	Mental	Communication	Multiple	Autism	Health	Behaviour or Emotion	Others
Turkey	Orthopaedic impairment	Hearing impairment	Visual impairment	- Moderate - Severe learning disability - Gifted or talented	Language and speech difficulty		Autism	Chronic illness		Neurological injury
United Kingdom (England)	Children with statements (records) of special educational needs									
United States	Orthopaedic impairments	Hearing impairments	Visual impairments	Mental retardation	Speech or language impairment	- Multiple disabilities - Deaf or blindness	Autism	Other health impairments		- Traumatic brain injury - Development delay

Starting from the analysis of these classifications, the LUDI Working Group 1 made some choices with respect to the following criteria:

- The need to adopt the most significant and useful categories for the project purposes: this means categories related to impairments that prevent children from playing freely
- The appropriateness of the terminology
- The need to avoid a proliferation of categories, rather to have broad categories with the possibility to indicate the severity of the impairment

The proposal for the LUDI Classification of disabilities[13] is reported in Table 4.2:

Table 4.2. LUDI Classification of disabilities

LUDI categories of disabilities
Mental or intellectual disability (mild, moderate, severe, profound)
Hearing impairments (partially hearing impaired – deaf)
Visual impairments (partially sighted – blind)
Communication disorders (language disorders)
Physical impairments (mild, moderate, severe)
Autism spectrum disorders
Multiple disabilities

4.3 Description of the LUDI Categories of Childhood Disabilities

The categories identified within the LUDI Classification of disabilities are described and defined as follows, by referring to two main international sources: the WHO International Statistical Classification of Diseases and Related Health Problems 10th Revision (ICD-10, 2010) and the Diagnostic and Statistical Manual of Mental Disorders 5th edition, published by the American Psychiatric Association (2013). Whenever

13 The LUDI categories of disabilities may also consider 'invisible disabilities' for project purposes. The term 'invisible' refers to disabilities that are less visible than other physical, sensory, or mobility impairments, and that are prevalent but commonly under recognised (Gaines et al., 2008; Missiuna et al., 2006). This category encompasses a heterogeneous group of major and minor neurodevelopmental disorders, attention deficit disorders, developmental coordination disorders, and specific learning disorders that may compromise play participation. While these conditions are defined in the Diagnostic and Statistical Manual of Mental Disorders 5th edition (APA, 2013), the affected children may be more subject to misconceptions regarding the legitimacy of their play difficulties and need of support to play. However, numerous researches have highlighted the need to be concerned by the consequences of neurodevelopmental disorder on children's playfulness and participation in play (Kennedy-Behr et al., 2013; Leipold & Bundy, 2000; Poulsen & Ziviani, 2004; Unhjem et al., 2014).

needed, reference will be also made to other sources and documents, because the two main documents aforementioned were not exhaustive for a functional description of all categories of childhood disabilities of LUDI.

4.3.1 Intellectual Disabilities

In the DSM-5, the neurodevelopmental disorders include three types of intellectual disabilities: the intellectual disability, the global developmental delay, and the unspecified intellectual disability. The intellectual disability should meet the following three criteria:

a) Deficits in intellectual functions: reasoning, problem-solving, planning, abstract thinking, judgement, academic learning, and experiential learning
b) Deficits in adaptive functioning involving three domains: conceptual, social, and practical, so that ongoing support is needed to meet the developmental and socio-cultural standards for personal independence and social responsibility; limits are related to one or more daily life activities, such as social participation, communication, independent living in several life contexts (home, school, work, and recreation)
c) Onset of intellectual and adaptive deficits during the infancy and childhood

The intellectual functioning is conventionally estimated through standardised and validated intelligence tests, and usually, a score lower than at least two standard deviations from the average represents a cognitive delay. The adaptive functioning is estimated by scales assessing social adaptation in a given environment. These measures provide an approximate indication of the degree of intellectual impairment. The diagnosis will also depend on the overall assessment of intellectual functioning by a skilled diagnostician.

Intellectual abilities and social adaptation may change over time, and, however poor, may improve as a result of training and rehabilitation. Diagnosis should be based on the current levels of functioning.

The DSM-5 includes the following levels of severity of the intellectual disability:

- Mild - Approximate IQ range of 55 to 70 (mental age from 8 to under 11 years). Likely to result in some learning difficulties in school. During adulthood, persons with mild intellectual impairment show social and occupational abilities that allow them to live autonomously, although they may need some degree of support.
- Moderate - Approximate IQ range of 40 to 55 (mental age from 4 to under 7 years). Likely to result in marked developmental delays in childhood, but most persons can learn to develop some degree of independence in self-care and acquire adequate communication and academic skills.
- Severe - Approximate IQ range of 25 to 40 (mental age from 18 months to under 4 years). Likely to result in continuous need of support.

- Profound - IQ under 25 (mental age below 18 months). Likely to result in severe limitation in self-care, continence, communication, and mobility.

4.3.2 Hearing Impairments

For the elaboration of the description in this category and the following – the visual impairments – two separate sources found on the Web have been used; the first is a document, the Kentucky's Office for the Americans with Disabilities Act, produced by the Kentucky Education and Workforce Development Cabinet[14]. The second source is located within the WHO website, in the section dedicated to the Media Centre, in particular in the 'Fact Sheet', in relation to the definition of deafness and hearing loss[15].

The hearing impairments are defined as a hearing loss that prevents a person from totally receiving sounds through the ear. There are four types of hearing losses:

- Conductive: Caused by diseases or obstructions in the outer or middle ear, which usually affect all frequencies of hearing. A hearing aid generally helps a person with a conductive hearing loss.
- Sensorineural: Results from damage to the inner ear. This loss can range from mild to profound, and often affects certain frequencies more than others. Sounds are often distorted, even with a hearing aid.
- Mixed: Occurs in both the inner and outer or middle ear.
- Central: Results from damage to the central nervous system.

Hearing loss may be mild, moderate, severe, or profound. It can affect one ear or both ears, and leads to difficulty in hearing conversational speech or loud sounds. 'Hard of hearing' refers to people with hearing loss ranging from mild to severe. They usually communicate through spoken language and can benefit from hearing aids, captioning, and assistive listening devices. People with more significant hearing losses may benefit from cochlear implants. 'Deaf' people mostly have profound hearing loss, which implies very little or no hearing.

4.3.3 Visual Impairments

Visual impairment is a functional limitation of the vision system, which cannot be recovered by usual means (glasses, for instance). It leads to loss of visual acuity, loss of visual field, visual distortion, or visual perception difficulties. Visual impairments

14 Retrieved from: http://www.ada.ky.gov/hearing_imp_def.htm.

15 Retrieved from: http://www.who.int/mediacentre/factsheets/fs300/en/.

range from partial to total loss of sight. Visual impairment is defined as a best-corrected visual acuity between 20/70 and 20/1200 (foot, accordingly to the Snellen chart, 1862), and blindness is defined as a visual acuity worse than 20/1200 with the best possible correction. There are four levels of visual impairments, according to the ICD-10:

- Mild visual impairment: Acuity equal to or better than 20/70.
- Moderate visual impairment: Acuity worse than 20/70 or equal to 20/200.
- Severe visual impairment: Acuity worse than 20/400 or equal to 20/1200.
- Blindness: Acuity worse than 20/1200.

The definition of 'legally blindness' varies from country to country. The assistance that a person with a visual impairment requires depends on the degree of sight loss and when the loss occurred. A person who is visually impaired may use magnifying glasses, enlarged print, or other strategies. A person who is legally blind relies more on the other senses to perceive the world, but still can be completely independent. This person may use a cane or a service dog, also called a 'guide dog'.[16]

4.3.4 Communication Disorders

This category is presented in the DSM-5 in the chapter on neurodevelopmental disorders, and includes deficits in language, speech, and communication. In particular, with regard to play and the aims of the project, only one category within communication disorders will be considered, that is the language disorder. The DSM-5 defines language as "the form, function, and use of a conventional system of symbols (i.e., spoken words, sign language, written words, pictures) in a rule-governed manner for communication" (2013: 41).

Language disorder is characterised by persistent difficulties in the acquisition and use of spoken, written, or sign language; deficits in comprehension or production include a reduced vocabulary, limited sentence structure, and impairments in discourse. The disorder emerged in early age and is not due to hearing, sensory, motor, or other neurological impairments. Language disorder affects communication, social participation, and occupational performances.

4.3.5 Physical Impairments

A physical impairment is permanent and substantially limits physical ability or motor skills. The physical capacity to move, coordinate actions, or perform physical activities

16 http://www.ada.ky.gov/vis_imp_def.htm.

is impaired, and the child faces challenges in one or more of the following areas: physical and motor tasks. independent movement, performing basic life functions.

Physical impairment can be either congenital or acquired. Children with congenital conditions are either born with physical difficulties or develop them soon after birth. Acquired disabilities are those developed through injury or disease while the child is developing normally. The age at which a condition develops often determines its impact on the child. Physical impairments can also be progressive or chronic. Physical impairments can be related to a problem to the performing system (skeleton, neuromuscular system, joints) or to the directive system (central nervous system), and in this last case, it can be specific or nonspecific.

Examples of impairments of the first type are muscular dystrophy, achondroplasia, juvenile rheumatoid arthritis, and so on; examples of the second type are cerebral palsy, ataxia, traumatic brain injury, neural tube defects, spinal cord injury, and so on.

Possible subdivisions (mild, moderate, severe) can be related to the physical extension of the impairment (i.e., number of limbs involved, presence of spasms or other forms of dyskinesia, extension and level of the neurologic injury, and so on). Unlike other categories and for intervention purposes, these subdivisions can be related to the extension of the needed support: slight support (mild); substantial support (moderate); very substantial support (severe).

4.3.6 Autism Spectrum Disorders

This category is included in the DSM-5 within the chapter on neurodevelopmental disorders, and can be identified through two main criteria:

a. Persistent deficits in social communication and social interaction across multiple contexts as manifested by the following: deficits in social-emotional reciprocity, deficits in nonverbal communicative behaviours used for social interaction, and deficits in developing, maintaining, and understanding relationships
b. Restricted, repetitive patterns of behaviour, interest, or activities as manifested by at least two of the following: stereotyped or repetitive motor movement, use of objects or speech; insistence on sameness; inflexible adherence to routines, or ritualised patterns of verbal or nonverbal behaviour; highly restricted, fixated interest that are abnormal in intensity or focus; and hyper or hyporeactivity to sensory input or unusual interest in sensory aspects of the environment

The severity specifiers may be used to describe the child's symptomatology with the recognition that severity may vary by context and fluctuate over time. Severity of social communication difficulties and restricted, repetitive behaviours should be separately rated.

Level 1 – Requiring support

- Social communication: Without support in place, deficits cause noticeable impairments: difficulty initiating social interactions, and clear examples of atypical or unsuccessful responses to social overtures of others are present; the child may appear to have decreased interest in social interactions.
- Restricted, repetitive behaviours: Inflexibility of behaviour causes insignificant interference with functioning in one or more contexts; difficulty in switching between activities. Problems of organisation and planning hamper independence.

Level 2 - Requiring substantial support

- Social communication: Marked deficits in verbal and nonverbal social communication skills; social impairments apparent even with supports in place; limited initiation of social interactions; reduced or abnormal responses to social overtures from others.
- Restricted, repetitive behaviours: Inflexibility of behaviour, difficulty coping with change, or other restricted or repetitive behaviours appear frequently enough to be obvious to the casual observer and interfere with functioning in a variety of contexts; distress and/or difficulty changing focus or action.

Level 3 - Requiring very substantial support

- Social communication: Severe deficits in verbal and nonverbal social communication skills cause severe impairments in functioning, very limited initiation of social interactions, and minimal response to social overtures from others.
- Restricted, repetitive behaviours: Inflexibility of behaviour, extreme difficulty coping with change, or other restricted or repetitive behaviours markedly interfere with functioning in all spheres; great distress and/or difficulty changing focus or action.

4.3.7 Multiple Disabilities

In literature, there is not an international consensus about the definition of multiple disabilities, because children with multiple disabilities show combination of concomitant impairments at physical, motor, intellectual, sensory, or communicative level.

The World Health Organisation defines a child with multiple impairments as a child with a significant physical disability combined with a sensory and/or cognitive disability (WHO, 1996:4). According to the Individuals with Disabilities Education Act (IDEA, U.S. Congress; 1975, 2004), a law by the U.S. Department of Education, the combination of multiple disabilities "causes such severe educational needs that cannot be accommodated in special education programs solely for one of the impairments". Thus, each child with multiple impairment shows a specific condition that can dramatically vary in respect to general intelligence, gross and fine motor skills, language, and social adaptation. Comorbidity with behavioural or psychological problems is common in children with multiple disabilities (Cadman et al., 1987).

According to the LUDI goal, which is to foster and guarantee play for the sake of play for disabled children, multiple disabilities are defined as a condition in which a sensory impairment is associated with another of the six disabilities listed before. In fact, the sensory channel is a fruitful mean to playfully interact with the child with disability and its damage brings additional challenges that need to be addressed and overcome.

References

American Psychiatric Association. (2013). *Diagnostic and statistical manual of mental disorders (DSM-5®)*. Arlington, VA: American Psychiatric Association Publishing.

Cadman, D., Boyle, M., Szatmari, P., & Offord, D. (1987) Chronic illness, disability, and mental and social well-being: Findings of the Ontario Child Health Study. *Paediatrics*, 79, 805-813.

Gaines, R., Missiuna, C., Egan, M., & McLean, J. (2008). Educational outreach and collaborative care enhances physician's perceived knowledge about Developmental Coordination Disorder. *BMC Health Services Research*, 8(1), 21.

Goodson, B. & Bronson, M. (1997). Which toy for which child. *Technical Report 285-286, U.S. Consumer Product Safety Commission*.

Kennedy-Behr, A., Rodger, S., & Mickan, S. (2013). A comparison of the play skills of preschool children with and without developmental coordination disorder. *OTJR: Occupation, Participation and Health*, 33(4), 198-208.

Leipold, E. E. & Bundy, A. (2000). Playfulness in children with attention deficit hyperactivity disorder. *Occupational Therapy Journal of Research*, 20(1), 61-82.

Missiuna, C., Gaines, R., & Soucie, H. (2006). Why every office needs a tennis ball: a new approach to assessing the clumsy child. *Canadian Medical Association Journal*, 175(5), 471-473.

Organization for Economic Cooperation and Development – Centre for Educational Research and Innovation (2007). *Students with Disabilities, Learning Difficulties and Disadvantages: Policies, Statistics and Indicators*. Retrieved from: http://www.oecd.org/edu/school/studentswithdisabilitieslearningdifficultiesanddisadvantagespoliciesstatisticsandindicators-2007edition.htm.

Poulsen, A. A., & Ziviani, J. M. (2004). Can I play too? Physical activity engagement of children with developmental coordination disorders. *Canadian Iournal of Occupational Therapy. Revue canadienne d'ergothérapie*, 71(2), 100.

Snellen, H. (1862). *Probebuchstaben zur Bestimmung der Sehschärfe*. Utrecht, NL: Van de Weijer.

Unhjem A., Eklund, K., & Nergard-Nilssen. (2014). Early communicative gestures and play as predictors of language development in children born with and without family risk for dyslexia. *Scandinavian Journal of Psychology*, 55, 326-332.

U.S. Congress (1975, 2004). *The Individuals with Disabilities Education Act–IDEA*. Retrieved from: http://www.parentcenterhub.org/repository/idea/.

United Nations (2006). *Convention on the Rights of Persons with Disabilities*. Retrieved from: http://www.un.org/disabilities/convention/conventionfull.shtml.
The United States National Institute of Play (unspecified date). *Pattern of play*. Retrieved from: http://www.nifplay.org/science/pattern-play.
World Health Organisation (2001). *International Classification of Functioning Disability and Health*. Geneva, CH: WHO.

Daniela Bulgarelli and Vaska Stancheva-Popkostadinova

5 Play in Children with Intellectual Disabilities

Intellectual disability (ID) is characterised by significantly below-average intellectual functioning and limitations in two or more areas of adaptive skills: communication, self-direction, social skills, self-care, personal independence at home or in community settings, school or work functioning, and maintenance of personal safety (Shalock et al., 2010).

Children with ID do not form a homogenous group (Brodin & Stancheva-Popkostadinova, 2009). The differences are based on the severity of intellectual disability (mild, moderate, severe, and profound) and comorbidity. The limitations in some adaptive skills often coexist with the strengths in other skills.

The biggest part of the children with ID face challenges in communication, emotion regulation, language, rapid processing of information, attention, executive functioning, and are more likely to show internalising and externalising problems.

5.1 Play in Children with ID

"The studies about medical and physical effects of different kinds of disability are predominant, and until the end of last century very little attention has been given to the way the nature of children's play is changed by a disability" (Webb, 2003:15).

Play in children with ID is studied from different perspectives: in comparison with children without ID (Blasco et al., 1993; Lieber, 1993; Malone, 2006); home settings versus school settings (Malone, 2009); correlations between specific psychological characteristics and particular types of play (Cunningham et al., 1985; Elias & Berk, 2002; Nader-Grosbois & Vieillevoye, 2012); role of parents in parent–child play interaction (Hauser-Cram & Howell, 2003; Roarch et al., 1998); parents' perceptions of children's play (Malone & Landers, 2001).

The severity of ID influences the nature and characteristics of children's play. Allen (1980) reported that play in children with ID may not emerge so naturally and informally as it does with other children, and may need to be encouraged. Comparing atypically and typically developing (TD) children, Hughes (2009) stressed that children with ID were more interested in the physical characteristics of play materials than in their representational possibilities; they were more likely to simply manipulate and handle play materials; they were more repetitive and less varied in toy play (Lender et al., 1988); finally, children were delayed in the emergence of symbolic play and were less likely to reach higher levels of sophistication.

In contrast with the previous positions, some studies by Malone et al. pointed out that the patterns of play in children with and without ID within the same context were similar: in fact, both groups of children spent nearly equal time in functional, constructive, and pretend play during home-based independent play situation (Malone, 2009; Malone & Stoneman, 1990). Moreover, Linn, Goodman, and Lender (2000) stated that despite the frequencies of passivity and repletion, children with ID spent the majority of their time engaging in spontaneous, nonrepetitive play. This picture also emerged in a study in which mothers' were requested to describe play in their children with ID (Malone & Landers, 2001).

5.2 Cognitive Play

With respect to the cognitive dimension of play, the development of play in children with ID proceeds similarly as for TD children; it is related to the child's level of cognitive functioning; thus, delays are usually present and symbolic play appears later (Beeghly, 1998; Cicchetti & Ganiban, 1990; Fewell et al., 1997; Gowen et al., 1992; Hill & McCune-Nicolich, 1981; Hughes, 2009; Libby et al., 1997; Motti et al., 1983; Turner & Small, 1985). Play of children with ID appears to be more repetitive than TD play because of distractibility and impairment in motivation, perception, learning (Lender et al., 1998; Morgenstern, 1968).

Messier, Ferland, and Majnemer (2008) reported that in a group of children with ID between 6 and 8 years of age, play age was about 2.5 years. Their practice play, involving gross and fine motor skills, their interest in sensory elements of play, and their interest in exploration were well-established, whereas all aspects related to imitation, imagination, and dramatisation abilities were delayed. Singh, Iacono, and Gray (2014) found that 12 two- to five-year-old children with Down Syndrome mainly performed functional play and less complex symbolic play. Thus, symbolic play typically appears later in children with ID (Hughes, 2009). Children with ID between 8 and 12 years of age displayed level of symbolic play similarly to TD children of similar mental age (3-6 years; Beeghly et al., 1989; Hill & McCune-Nicholic, 1981; Motti et al., 1983; Nader-Grosbois & Vieillevoye, 2012). When involved in structured situation, in which, for instance, play objectives are defined by adults, children with ID showed higher pretend play level (Nader-Grosbois & Vieillevoye, 2012). In terms of their play with objects, children with ID seem to prefer structured materials, such as puzzles and jacks, while typical children of the same mental age prefer open-ended materials (e.g., art supplies) that allow them to be creative and imaginative.

In literature, studies on practice and symbolic play in children with ID are present, mainly because these are intended as indicators of cognitive development. On the other hand, studies about constructive and rule play in this population are uncommon because of children with IDs' difficulty in cognitive reasoning, planning of strategies and goals, and so on. In general, children with ID are less likely than other children to combine objects appropriately in play (Hughes, 2009).

It is worth noticing that children with IDs ludic attitude, consisting curiosity, initiative, pleasure, spontaneity, and participation, were found to not being related to the IQ level and cognitive functioning (Linn et al., 2000; Luttropp & Granlund, 2010; Messier et al., 2008).

5.3 Social Play

With respect to the social dimension of play, compared to the TD children, children with ID show higher proportion of solitary play (Guralnick et al., 1996b; Guralnick & Groom, 1987a; 1987b; Kopp et al., 1992), interact less with peers, and exhibit lower levels of complexity in engagement (Guralnick et al., 2006; Luttropp & Granlund, 2010). Moreover, they have specific problems in ludic interactions, above all, with peers. In general, social interactions are more restricted than those of comparable groups of children (Guralnick, 1997), and children with ID are less likely to initiate play with peers and have difficulties with cooperation (Luttropp & Granlund, 2010; Messier et al., 2008).

In fact, playing with peers is a high-demanding activity from a linguistic, cognitive, and social point of view: it implies self-regulatory strategies, achieving interpersonal goals, sustaining and coordinating play sequences, resolving conflicts, processing complex social information, and so on (Guralnick 1999a; Luttropp & Granlund, 2010; Vieillevoye & Nader-Grosbois, 2008). Consequently, with difficulties in complex interactions, children with ID have been found to be more socially included during structured activities in kindergartens (Luttropp & Granlund, 2010).

Because of these difficulties, during ludic interaction, children with ID also spent more time in passivity, or disengagement from activity than TD children (Krakow & Kopp, 1982, 1983; Lender et al., 1998; Linn et al., 2000). In these children, passive behaviours increased according to the amount of time spent in playing. Moreover, while TD children can quickly coordinate and alternate play and social interaction with the partner, children with ID need to stop playing to interact with the partner, thus reducing the total amount of ludic interactions (Linn et al., 2000).

Children with ID have smaller social networks than TD children and rarely have best friends to play with frequently. Thus, they spend higher percentage of their social activities (including play) with adults (parents, teachers, educators) or siblings, who are more likely to adapt themselves to the cognitive and interactional level of the children with ID and can better understand their communication (de Falco et al., 2008; Luttropp & Granlund, 2010; Moyson & Roeyers, 2012; Solish et al., 2010). Moreover, it could be difficult for TD children to understand and anticipate the reaction of children with ID, because of their difficulties in complex social interactions and in self-regulation (Ytterhus, 2003), whereas siblings, for instance, can better interpret children with ID communication and behaviour (Moyson & Roeyers, 2012).

IDs influence others' behaviours and specifically parental support during play sessions. For instance, mothers of children with ID tend to be more directive and supportive than mothers of TD children (Hauser-Cram & Howell, 2003; Roarch et al., 1998). This style was functional to support children's play: in fact, it was associated with more object play and vocalisation by children with ID (Roarch et al., 1998). It is worth noticing that among children with ID, great individual differences emerged: degree and type of disability were not strongly correlated with the child's social competence and participation (Luttropp & Granlund, 2010).

5.4 Conclusion

The literature about play in children with ID covered more than 45 years of research and still this topic is of current interest. Some studies compared play in children with and without disabilities, others presented specific aspects of play, or play in specific disability groups.

Even if there are some controversial results, majority of the studies showed that there are more similarities than differences in play of children with ID and without ID. Despite some individual differences, both the cognitive and social complexities of play displayed by children with ID are mostly related to the development of their cognitive and social competences. Thus, supportive environments and supportive partners are important to give children with ID a chance to play for the sake of play.

References

Allen, K. E. (1980). Mainstreaming: What we have learned? *Young Children*. 35(5), 54-63.

Beeghly, M. (1998). Emergence of symbolic play: Perspectives from typical and atypical development. In J. A., Burack, R. M., Hodapp, & Zigler, E. (Eds). *Handbook of mental retardation and development*, (pp. 240-289). Cambridge, UK: Cambridge University Press.

Beeghly, M., Perry, B. W., & Cicchetti, D. (1989). Structural and affective dimensions of play development in young children with Down syndrome. *International Journal of Behavioural Development*, *12*(2), 257-277.

Blasco, P. M., Bailey, D. B., & Burchinal, M. A. (1993). Dimensions of mastery in same-age and mixed-age integrated classrooms. *Early Childhood Research Quarterly*, *8*(2), 193-206.

Brodin, J., & Stancheva-Popkostadinova, V. (2009). Early interventions in children with intellectual disabilities. *Annual of Union of Scientists: Science, Culture and Education*, *3rd volume*, 215-220.

Cicchetti, D., & Ganiban, J. (1990). The organization and coherence of developmental processes in the infants and children with Down syndrome. In R. M. Hodapp, J. A Burack, & E. Zigler, Eds. *Issues in the developmental approach to mental retardation* (pp. 169-225). Cambridge, UK: Cambridge University Press.

Cunningham, C. C., Glenn, S. M., Wilkinson, P., & Sloper, P. (1985). Mental ability, symbolic play and receptive and expressive language of young children with Down's syndrome. *Journal of Child Psychology and Psychiatry*, *26*(2), 255-265.

De Falco, S., Esposito, G., Venuti, P., & Bornstein, M. H. (2008). Fathers' play with their Down syndrome children. *Journal of Intellectual Disability Research*, *52*(6), 490-502.

Elias, C. L., & Berk, L. E. (2002). Self-regulation in young children: Is there a role for sociodramatic play?. *Early Childhood Research Quarterly*, *17*(2), 216-238.

Fewell, R., T. Ogura, A. Wheeden (1997). The Relationship Between Play and Communication Skills in Young Children with Down Syndrome. *Topics in Early Childhood Special Education*. *17*(1), 103-118.

Gowen, J. W., Johnson-Martin, N., Goldman, B. D., & Hussey, B. (1992). Object play and exploration in children with and without disabilities: a longitudinal study. *American journal of mental retardation*, *97*(1), 21-38.

Guralnick, M. J. (1999a). Family and child influences on the peer-related social competence of young children with developmental delays. *Mental Retardation and Developmental Disabilities Research Reviews*, *5*, 21–29.

Guralnick, M. J. (2006). Peer relationships and the mental health of young children with intellectual delays. *Journal of Policy and Practice in Intellectual Disabilities*, *3*(1), 49-56.

Guralnick, M. J., Connor, R. T., Neville, B., & Hammond, M. A. (2006). Promoting the peer-related social development of young children with mild developmental delays: Effectiveness of a comprehensive intervention. *American Journal on Mental Retardation, 111(5)*, 336-356.

Guralnick, M. J., & Groom, J. M. (1985). Correlates of peer related social competence in developmentally delayed preschool children. *American Journal of Mental Deficiency*, *90*, 140–150.

Guralnick, M. J., & Groom, J. M. (1987a). The peer relations of mildly delayed and nonhandicapped preschool children in mainstreamed playgroups. *Child Development*, *58*, 1556–1572.

Hauser-Cram, P., & Howell, A. (2003). The development of young children with disabilities and their families: Implications for policies and programs. In R. M. Lerner, F. Jacobs, & D. Wertlieb (Eds.), *Handbook of applied developmental science, Vol. 1* . Thousand Oaks, CA: Sage, 259-279.

Hill, P. M., & McCune-Nicolich, L. (1981). Pretend play and patterns of cognition in Down's syndrome children. *Child Development, 52*, 611–617.

Hughes, F. (2009). Play In Special Populations. In: F. Hughes (Ed.), *Children, Play, and Development*. London, UK: SAGE Publications (pp. 183-210).

Krakow, J. B., & Kopp, C. B. (1982). Sustained attention in young Down syndrome children. *Topics in Early Childhood Education, 2*, 32–42.

Krakow, J. B., & Kopp, C. B. (1983). The effects of developmental delay on sustained attention in young children. *Child Development, 54*(5), 1143–1155.

Lender, W. L., Goodman, J. F., & Linn, M. I. (1998). Repetitive activity in the play of children with mental retardation. *Journal of Early Intervention*, *21*(4), 308–322.

Libby, S., Powell, S., Messer, D., & Jordan, R. (1997). Imitation of pretend play acts by children with autism and Down syndrome. *Journal of Autism and Developmental Disorders*, *27*(4), 365–383.

Lieber, J. (1993). A comparison of social pretend play in young children with and without disabilities. *Early Education and Development*, *4*(3), 148–161.

Linn, M. I., Goodman, J. F., & Lender, W. L. (2000). Played out? Passive behavior by children with Down syndrome during unstructured play. *Journal of Early Intervention*, *23*(4), 264–278.

Luttropp, A., & Granlund, M. (2010). Interaction–it depends–a comparative study of interaction in preschools between children with intellectual disability and children with typical development. *Scandinavian Journal of Disability Research*, *12*(3), 151–164.

Malone, D. M. (2006). Contextually influenced patterns of play-developmental age associations for preschoolers with and without mental retardation. *Early Childhood Education Journal*, *34*(3), 215–225.

Malone, M. (2009). Patterns of Home- and Classroom-based Toy Play of Preschoolers With and Without Intellectual Disabilities. *International Journal of Disability, Development and Education*. *56*(4), 333–347.

Malone, D., & Landers, M. (2001). Mothers' Perceptions of the Toy Play of Preschoolers with Intellectual Disabilities. *International Journal of Disability, Development and Education*, *48*(1), 91–102.

Messier, J., Ferland, F., & Majnemer, A. (2008). Play behavior of school age children with intellectual disability: Their capacities, interests and attitude. *Journal of Developmental and Physical Disabilities*, *20*(2), 193–207.

Morgenstern, F. S. (1968). Psychological Handicaps in the Play of Handicapped Children. *Developmental Medicine & Child Neurology*, *10*(1), 115–120.

Motti, F., Cicchetti, D., & Sroufe, L. A. (1983). From infant affect expression to symbolic play: The coherence of development in Down syndrome children. *Child Development*, *54*(5), 1168–1175.

Moyson, T., & Roeyers, H. (2012). 'The overall quality of my life as a sibling is all right, but of course, it could always be better'. Quality of life of siblings of children with intellectual disability: the siblings' perspectives. *Journal of Intellectual Disability Research*, *56*(1), 87–101.

Nader-Grosbois, N., & Vieillevoye, S. (2012). Variability of self-regulatory strategies in children with intellectual disability and typically developing children in pretend play situations. *Journal of Intellectual Disability Research*. *56*(2), 140–156.

Roach, M. A., Barratt, M. S., Miller, J. F., & Leavitt, L. A. (1998). The structure of mother–child play: Young children with Down syndrome and typically developing children. *Developmental Psychology*, *34*(1), 77–87.

Schalock, R. L., Borthwick-Duffy, S. A., Bradley, V. J., Buntinx, W. H., Coulter, D. L., Craig, E. M., ... & Shogren, K. A. (2010). *Intellectual disability: Definition, classification, and systems of supports*. Washington, DC: American Association on Intellectual and Developmental Disabilities.

Singh, S. J., Iacono, T., & Gray, K. M. (2014). An Investigation of the Intentional Communication and Symbolic Play Skills of Children With Down Syndrome and Cerebral Palsy in Malaysia. *Journal of Early Intervention*, 36(*2*), 71–89.

Solish, A., Perry, A., & Minnes, P. (2010). Participation of children with and without disabilities in social, recreational and leisure activities. *Journal of Applied Research in Intellectual Disabilities*, *23*(3), 226–236.

Turner, I. F., & Small, J. D. (1985). Similarities and differences in behaviour between mentally handicapped and normal preschool children during play. *Child: care, health and development*, *11*(6), 391–401.

Vieillevoye, S., & Nader-Grosbois, N. (2008). Self-regulation during pretend play in children with intellectual disability and in normally developing children. *Research in Developmental Disabilities, 29*(3), 256-272.

Webb, R. (2003). Public play provision for children with disabilities. *Bray, Ireland: Sudgradh*. Retrieved from: http://sugradh.org/news/sugradh_RP0301.pdf.

Ytterhus, B. (2003). *Barns sociala samvaro. Inklusion och exclusion i fo¨rskolan* [Social togetherness for children. Inclusion and exclusion in preschool]. Lund, S: Studentlitteratur.

Anna Andreeva, Pietro Celo, Nicole Vian

6 Play in Children with Hearing Impairments

According to the World Health Organisation (WHO, 2015), 32 million children worldwide have hearing loss. The degree of hearing loss is classified into four subgroups: mild (26–40 dB), moderate (41–60 dB), severe (61–80 dB), and profound (over 80 dB) (WHO, 2015). The presence of hearing loss in childhood puts a child at risk for language, social, and academic difficulties. It can negatively affect the quality of life, even if the hearing loss is mild (Burkey, 2006). Language development and modalities of communication are strictly related to the emergence of play skills and influence the relationship with other children in mutual play situations.

Many factors affect the communication skills, as well as the cognitive and also the play development of children with hearing loss. They include: the degree of hearing loss, its etiology, the audiometric configuration, the age of onset, the age at which the child's hearing impairment is identified, the adequacy and the type of programme in the rehabilitation intervention, the presence of other impairments, the consistency of the adopted amplification mode (hearing aid, cochlear implant, bone-anchored hearing aid), the family and environmental influences and the attitudes of the other children and their parents (Spencer & Marschark, 2010; Sininger et al., 2010; Paul & Whitelaw, 2011; Harris, 2014; Mills et al., 2014).

6.1 Play and Language Development in Children with Hearing Impairments

Young children explore the surrounding world through play: it is very important for a child's development. Play has been recognised by the United Nations High Commission for Human Rights as a right of every child. Play is crucial for communication, cognitive, physical, social, and emotional development of young children (Ginsburg, 2007).

Many studies have explored play in groups of children with hearing impairment. A hearing-impaired child can be as competent as a typically developing one. Individuals with hearing loss necessarily play, think, learn, or behave exactly like their hearing peers. Some research compared play behaviour of children with and without hearing impairment; part of the studies found similarities, but others ascertained differences that were strongly associated with language levels (Higginbotham & Baker, 1981 in Schirmer, 1989; Spencer & Marschark, 2010).

Hearing-impaired children and their families have a variety of opportunities to choose the communication methods as well as the rehabilitation methodology that will support learning. Usually, parents of children with mild or moderate hearing loss choose oral approaches (i.e., listening and spoken language), whereas for children with more severe hearing losses, parents may opt for a sign language. Other functional outcomes, such as later socialisation, academic achievement, and self-esteem, are also considered by parents when deciding on the communication mode (Harris, 2014).

The interval between birth and auditory rehabilitation is not always negatively correlated with the neural development (Kral, 2013), as well as play, perceptual, linguistic, and cognitive abilities (Geers et al., 2007; Pisoni et al., 2008; Peterson et al., 2010; Havy et al., 2013). In cases of early identification of hearing loss, the communicative functions and play are not compromised in deaf children as well as in those children exposed to deaf sign language or in situations of bilingualism (Grosjean, 2015). Evidently, if detected language skills are related to oral skills, most of the deaf children will be out of compliance with the standard. In fact, bilingual children in inclusive school showed cognitive levels and language skills in sign language similar to hearing children (Tommasuolo, 2006).

It is worth noticing that the condition of a deaf child born in a family of deaf parents and then genetically close to them is different from that of many deaf children born to hearing parents. Congenital or acquired hearing impairment puts the child in a situation of diversity about their family, and this determines the approach to rehabilitation methods. In case one or both parents of the child are deaf and use the sign language, they usually find it very natural to adopt the sign language for the communication exchanges with their child.

What is important about language and play development is not the degree of hearing loss, but sharing the same condition and the same way of being in the world. Indeed, any communication delay does not seem to be given by deafness as such, but by the failure of early communicative interaction between adults and the deaf child (Malfatti, 2009). The lack of a real communicative relationship affects play more than the type of hearing impairment or the type of family.

White and White (1987) studied a group of young children with severe to profound hearing loss. They explored the relation between the child's age at the beginning of intervention, the hearing status of the family (deaf versus hearing parents), and the outcomes in language development. Children born in families with deaf parents were identified rather early because of routine hearing screening for infants. This situation gave the chance for these infants to begin early with the intervention and rehabilitation. This study found that the early identification and intervention could be a predictor of better spoken language in these children (Sininger et al., 2010), and correspondingly, of better play development. Today newborn hearing screening and cochlear implants give the opportunity for more children to rely on spoken language from an early age. When the level of verbal communication in children with hearing impairment is similar to their hearing peers, they have equal abilities to interact in play.

6.2 Play between Parents and Children with Hearing Impairments

Parents are the first playmates of children, because of their response to the playful infant behaviour. Infants naturally engage in different forms of play activities. During the years they grow up and have more experiences, thanks to interactions with adults and peers. It is their play with objects and people that stimulates brain development, and subsequently, cognitive growth (Piaget, 1962). One of the earliest forms of infant play is the repetitive motor activity. Infants also play by making sounds. They find these vocalisations pleasurable, and also draw attention and provoke playful response from caregivers (Wellhousen, 2002). Children with hearing impairment naturally produce rhythmic motor play through vocalisations, but this production decreases because they cannot hear themselves and cannot feel pleasure in listening to their own babbling. But, in case of consistent use of proper amplification (hearing aid, cochlear implant, bone-anchored hearing aid), the hearing abilities are stimulated, and respectively, they have a positive effect on the child–parent interaction and play behaviour.

Joint attention between a parent and a child develops during the first three years of life. This developmental process facilitates the acquisition of new words through interpersonal interactions and play. Joint attention subsequently forms representational skills and use of symbols in play. Cejas et al. (2014) found that young deaf children of hearing parents, compared to hearing counterparts, have deficits in joint engagement, which are related to oral language. In the youngest age groups, deaf children spend more time in unengaged states and less time in symbol states (e.g., parent and child are taking turns pretending to feed a doll). Clearly, the focus of their research is on oral relation and does not take into account shared communication in sign language. These results contrast with those from a study done by Spencer and Waxman (1995), which showed no differences in engagement states in play between deaf and hearing children aged 9 to 18 months.

6.3 Pretend Play in Children with Hearing Impairments

Researches about pretend play reported no significant differences comparing children with typical development and hearing-impaired children (Lyon, 1997; Spencer & Deyo, 1993; Spencer, 1996 in Brown et al., 2001). In 1990, Spencer, Deyo and Grindstaff showed that deaf children with deaf parents, who use sign language as their first language to communicate, spent equivalent amount of time in pretend play and produced the same amount and level of pretend play as their hearing counterparts. Another research by Brown et al. (2001) reported about pretend play and language production in children with hearing loss (between 3 and 6 years). The study showed that deaf children who have significant spoken language delay engaged in pretend play less often than their hearing peers (Higginbotham & Baker, 1981; Schirmer, 1989;

Cornelius & Hornett, 1990; Brown et al., 1997; Selmi & Rueda, 1998: in Brown et al., 2001). The scores for each one of the structures underpinning pretend play were lower in children with hearing loss. Children with hearing loss between 12 and 30 months of age in oral programmes produced lesser imaginative play than their hearing peers. Differences between the experimental and control groups were found in the language domain, but not in the cognitive domain (Brown et al., 2001). Verbal communication of hearing-impaired children is affected, but the nonverbal communication and time spent in pretend play are similar to typically developing children.

6.4 Symbolic Play in Children with Hearing Impairments

Humans use a wide variety of symbolic systems—spoken language, reading and writing, numbers, painting, drawing, music, and so on. Children develop these systems during the first five years of life by learning during play. Normally, play with language starts under the age of one, playing with sounds of the language or languages children are hearing around them. This is a very active process and quickly develops into making up new words, playing with rhymes. In case of hearing loss at an early age, it would result in oral language delay and the symbolic play would be affected.

Slade (1994) quotes a longitudinal study of play in six deaf children aged 1–3 by Gregory and Mogford (1983) who found that children with hearing impairment clearly demonstrated the capacity to use objects symbolically. But, comparing to the hearing counterparts of the same age, deaf children did not enact sequences of similar length and complexity (Slade & Wolf, 1994).

6.5 Free Play in Children with Hearing Impairments

Play provides a context in which children are motivated to communicate, and the availability of playmates increases the frequency and range of opportunities for language practice. Initiating, mediating, and sustaining a joint, playful activity requires children to use language in innovative ways and challenge them to communicate more clearly in social exchanges. Mills et al.'s (2014) findings in a study are supported by Odom et al. (1993). They observed that verbal interactions between peers were more likely to occur during play than during any other classroom activity. Barton and Wolery (2008) found that providing an intervention to increase play skills led to increased vocalisations, even though language was not a direct target of the intervention (Mills et al., 2014). It seems that free play supports language development of young children.

Play could be an effective medium for developing the necessary relationship to foster appropriate interaction (e.g., play turn-taking, sharing), and ultimately social communicative growth (e.g., vocal/verbal initiations, responding, and turn-taking) between children with and without hearing loss (Bat-Chava & Deignan, 2001). The magnitude of language skills essential for spontaneous play is considerable.

De Luzio and Girolametto (2011) evaluated the types of initiations and responses during play between children with normal hearing and children with severe to profound hearing loss. They found no significant difference between the two groups in terms of their initiation efforts. Both deaf and hearing preschoolers frequently used vocalisations, smiles, and object-related acts as strategies to initiate play (Vandell & George, 1981). Hearing-impaired children used similar initiation strategies as their hearing peers. They include nonverbal initiation, invitation to play, offering an object, or imitating the behaviour of other children (Weisel et al., 2005).

Play behaviour in preschoolers with and without hearing loss was described in several research articles. Harris (2014) quotes a study by Lederberg et al. (1987) about free play, in which researchers documented the duration, the number, and the complexity of children's interactions. The conclusion of the study was that, during free play, both hearing and hearing-impaired children interacted more frequently with peers with similar hearing abilities (Harris, 2014).

6.6 Social Play in Children with Hearing Impairments

A study of play in nursery school by Schvarfman (1977) found differences in quality and nature of play between hearing-impaired and typically developing children. Deaf children spent more of their time as onlookers and in solitary play. They engaged in less parallel play and in less cooperative and dramatic play with their hearing peers (Slade, 1994).

Qayyum, Khan, and Rais (2015) observed play behaviour during leisure time of children with hearing impairment in special schools. They found that the most frequent play behaviour was social play (group play) followed by non-play behaviour (active conversation) and the last was cognitive play (games with rules). The cognitive functional play was the least because these games require better understanding of rules through listening. Qayyum et al. found that games, which require listening to rules before start of play, were not understood well by the children with hearing impairment. Pupils played better games that only require visual cues (Qayyum et al., 2015).

Xie (2013) quotes a research by Anita and Dittillo (1998) focused on social play of children with hearing impairment and hearing children during inside play in a small group. They found that children with hearing impairment engaged in significantly less associative or cooperative play than children with normal hearing, but they engaged equally in non-play and social play.

6.7 Conclusion

Many researchers explore play in hearing-impaired children. They found a strong relationship between play and language development. Play and language are indirectly influenced by the hearing status and the modality of communication (sign language or spoken language). Less optimal early experiences, such as deprivation of linguistic stimuli by the caregiver, lack of exposure to sign language, linguistics re-education delay, could impede normal cognitive and linguistic development of hearing-impaired children. Better language development in both sign language and spoken language is a predictor of better play behaviour. Children with hearing impairment think, learn, play, and behave exactly like their hearing peers. Deaf children could need more visual signs, cues, or speech reading and those need more time in turn-taking exchanges. However, more time in the exchanges does not mean worse quality of play interaction, especially when this is made with suitable communication mode for each child with hearing impairment. If the children with hearing loss are provided with supportive communication from early stage of their life, they develop and play like typically developing children.

References

Antia, S. D., & Dittillo, D. A. (1998). A comparison of the peer social behavior of children who are Deaf/Hard of Hearing and Hearing. *Journal of Children's Communication Development*, 19, 1-10.

Barton, E. E., & Wolery, M. (2008). Teaching pretend play to children with disabilities: A review of the literature. *Topics in Early Childhood Special Education*, 28, 109-125.

Bat-Chava, Y., Deignan, E. (2001). Peer relationships of children with cochlear implants. *Journal of Deaf Studies and Deaf Education*, 6(3).

Brown, P. M., Prescott, S. J., Rickards, F. W. & Paterson, M. M. (1997). Communicating about pretend play: A comparison of the utterance of four year old normally hearing and hearing-impaired children in an integrated kindergarten. *Volta Review*, 99(1), 5-17.

Brown, P. M., Rickards, F.W., Bortoli, A. (2001). Structures Underpinning Pretend Play and Word Production in Young Hearing Children and Children with Hearing Loss. *Journal of Deaf Studies and Deaf Education*, 6(1).

Burkey, J. M. (2006). *Baby Boomers and Hearing Loss: a Guide to Prevention and Care*. New Brunswick, NJ: Rutgers University Press.

Cejas, I., Barker, D. H., Quittner, A. L., Niparko, J. K. (2014). Development of Joint Engagement in Young Deaf and Hearing Children: Effects of Chronological Age and Language Skills. *Journal of Speech, Language, and Hearing Research*, 57, 1831-1841.

Cornelius, G., & Hornett, D. (1990). The play behavior of hearing-impaired kindergarten children. *American Annals of the Deaf*, 135(4), 316-321.

De Luzio, J., & Girolametto, L. (2011). Peer interactions of preschool children with and without hearing loss. *Journal of Speech, Language, and Hearing Research*, 54(4), 1197-1210.

Geers A. E., Nicholas J. G., Moog J. S. (2007). Estimating the influence of cochlear implantation on language development in children. *Audiological Medicine*, 5, 262-273.

Ginsburg, K. R. (2007). The importance of play in promoting healthy child development and maintaining strong parent-child bonds. *Paediatrics*, 119(1), 182-191.

Gregory, S., & Mogford, K. (1983). The Development of Symbolic Play in Young Deaf Children. In A. Slade, & P. D. Wolf (Eds.), *Children at Play: Clinical and Developmental Approaches to Meaning and Representation*. New York and Oxford: Oxford University Press.
Grosjean, F. (2015). *Parler plusieurs langues: Le monde des bilingues* [Speaking several languages: The world of bilingualism]. Paris, F: Albin Michel.
Harris, L.G. (2014). *Social-Emotional Development in Children with Hearing Loss*. Theses and Dissertations-Communication Sciences and Disorders. Paper 4.
Havy, M., Nazzi T., & Bertoncini J. (2013). Phonetic processing during the acquisition of new words in 3-to-6 year-old-French-speaking deaf children with cochlear implants. *Journal of Communication Disorders*. 46, 181-192.
Higginbotham, D. J., & Baker, B. M. (1981). Social participation and cognitive play differences in hearing-impaired and normally hearing preschoolers. *Volta Review*, 83, 135-149.
Kral, A. (2013). Auditory critical periods: a review from system's perspective. *Neuroscience*, 247, 117-133.
Lyon, M. E., (1997). Symbolic play and language development in young deaf children. *Deafness and Education*, 21(2), 10-20.
Malfatti, M. (2009) *La comprensione sociale del bambino sordo nella scuola dell'infanzia: relazione educativa con l'insegnante e abilità di mentalizzazione* [Social understanding of the deaf child in kindergarten: educational relationship with the teacher and mentalization ability]. Ph.D. Thesis. Università degli Studi Roma Tre.
Mills, P. E., Beecher, C. C., Dale, Ph. S., Cole, K. N., & Jenkins, J. R. (2014). Language of Children with Disabilities to Peers at Play: Impact of Ecology. *Journal of Early Intervention*, 36(2), 111-130.
Odom, S. L., McConnell, S. R., & Chandler, L. K. (1993). Acceptability and feasibility of classroom-based social interaction interventions for young children with disabilities. *Exceptional Children*, 60, 226-236.
Piaget, J. (1962). *Play, Dreams, and Imitation in Childhood*. New York, NY: W.W. Norton & Co.
Peterson N. R., Pisoni D. B., & Miyamotoa R. T. (2010). Cochlear implants and spoken language processing abilities: review and assessment of the literature. *Restorative Neurology and Neuroscience*, 28, 237-250.
Pisoni D. B., Conway C. M., Kronenberger W. G., Horn D. L., Karpicke J., & Henning S. C. (2008). Efficacy and effectiveness of cochlear implants in deaf children. In: M. Marschark, & P. Hauser (Eds.), *Deaf Cognition: Foundations and Outcomes* (pp. 52-101). New York, NY: Oxford University Press.
Qayyum, A., Khan, A. Z., & Rais, R. A. (2015). Exploring play of children with sensory impairments in special schools at Karachi, Pakistan. *The Qualitative Report*, 20(2), 1-17.
Schirmer, B. R. (1989). Relationship between imaginative play and language development in hearing-impaired children. *American Annals of the Deaf*, 134(3), 219-222.
Selmi, A. M., & Rueda, R. S. (1998). A naturalistic study of collaborative play transformations of preschoolers with hearing impairment. *Journal of Early Intervention*, 27(4), 299-307.
Sininger, Y. S., Grimes, A., & Christensen, E. (2010). Auditory development in early amplified children: Factors influencing auditory-based communication outcomes in children with hearing loss. [Research Support, N.I.H., Extramural]. *Ear and Hearing*, 31(2), 166-185.
Slade, A. & Wolf, P. D. (1994). *Children at Play: Clinical and Developmental Approaches to Meaning and Representation*. New York and Oxford: Oxford University Press.
Spencer, P. & Waxman, S. (1995). Joint Attention and Maternal Attention Strategies: 9, 12 & 18 months. In *Maternal responsiveness and child competency in deaf and hearing children*. Final Report. Grant H023C10077, OSERS, US. Department of Education.
Spencer, P. E. (1996). The association between language and symbolic play at two years: Evidence from deaf toddlers. *Child Development*, 67, 867-876.

Spencer, P. E., & Deyo, D. (1993). Cognitive and social aspects of deaf children's play. In M. Marschark, & M. D. Clark (Eds.), *Psychological perspectives on deafness* (pp. 65-91). Hillsdale, NJ: Lawrence Erlbaum.

Spencer, P. E., Deyo, D., & Grindstaff, N. (1990). Symbolic play behaviour of hearing impaired and hearing toddlers. In: D. F. Moores, & K. P. Meadow-Orleans (Eds.), *Educational and Developmental Aspects of Hearing Impairment.* Washington, DC: Gallaudet University Press.

Spencer, P. E., & Marschark, M. (2010). *Evidence-Based Practice in educating Deaf and Hard-of-Hearing Students.* New York, NY: Oxford University Press.

Tommasuolo, E. (2006). *La valutazione delle abilità linguistiche in bambini e ragazzi sordi* [Evaluation of linguistic abilities in deaf children]. Ph.D. Thesis. Università degli Studi di Roma La Sapienza, Roma.

Vandell, D. L., & George, L. (1981). Social interaction in hearing and deaf preschoolers: Successes and failures in initiations. *Child Development*, 52, 627-635.

Weisel, A., Most, T., & Efron, C. (2005). Initiations of social interactions by young hearing impaired preschoolers. *Journal of Deaf Studies and Deaf Education*, 10, 161-170.

Wellhousen, K. (2002). *Outdoor Play, Every Day: Innovative Play Concepts for Early Childhood.* Delmar, UK: Cengage Learning.

White, S. J., & White, R. E. C. (1987). The effects of hearing status of the family and age of intervention on receptive and expressive oral language skills in hearing impaired infants. *Monographs of the American Speech, Language and Hearing Association*, 26, 9-24.

World Health Organisation (2015). *Grades of Hearing Impairment.* Retrieved from: http://www.who.int/pbd/deafness/hearing_impairment_grades/en/.

Xie, Y. (2013). Peer Interaction of Children with Hearing Impairment. *International Journal of Psychological Studies*; 5, 17-25.

Mira Tzvetkova-Arsova and Tamara Zappaterra

7 Play in Children with Visual Impairments

7.1 Basic Issues on Play in Children with Visual Impairments

As mentioned in Chapter 1, "play is a range of voluntary, intrinsically motivated activities normally associated with recreational pleasure and enjoyment" (Garvey, 1990). Play is also the child's main 'job'. It is often associated mainly with its visual aspects–looking at the toys, and thus, playing with them, seeing the play-partners, and initiating a game together, or in other words, engaging in the play activity through establishing a visual control, visual collaboration, and visual participation.

Many researches have been dedicated to play in children with visual impairments; within these studies, comparison are often offered, with respect to play, among the groups of blind, low-vision, and sighted children. Most of them conclude that visually impaired children, in general, experience major challenges and delays in many developmental areas, including play. According to Lowenfeld (1948), for instance, the limits of blind children are situated in the following three main areas:

a. In the control of the environment and the self in relation to it.
b. In the ability to get about.
c. In the range and variety of concepts.

Other researchers (Rowland, 1985) report that the delays and limitations experienced by visually impaired children and adults may include:

a. Sensory delay.
b. Social delay (difficulties in the quality and quantity of social relations).
c. Political delay (limits in the political and social awareness that their condition must be protected with egalitarian rights).

On the other hand, studies revealed that visually impaired children and sighted children have equal levels of development in many other areas, such as:

- Language development (Kirk & Gallaghar, 1979)
- Cognitive development and the intellectual abilities (Bateman, 1963; Litvak, 1985).
- School achievements (Gomulicki, 1961).

The famous blind Italian educator Augusto Romagnoli indicates that the blind child acquires through play the awareness of self, of the others and of their otherness, experiences solidarity and cooperation. So, play must be pursued as a principle of maximum socialisation (Romagnoli, 1924).

Based on these findings, one may expect that play is also delayed or compromised in blind and low-vision children. Different studies confirm this assumption. For instance, a Nordic study about five-year-old children in kindergartens identified four separate behaviour patterns (Sommer, 2003):

a) Social interactive behaviour. The child:
- is able to focus his or her attention on and follow the intentions of other children;
- is able to mark and follow his or her intentions, ideas, and desires – but is also able to adapt them to the interests of other children;
- is able to interpret and size up the intentions and enterprises of other children;
- is able to act in order to facilitate that his or her intentions and enterprises are carried out;
- is often able to leave his or her mark on the mutual interaction in the group in a positive way through his or her intentions, initiatives, and enterprises;
- is characterised as well integrated in the group of children.

b) Self-marking behaviour. The child:
is characterised by a strong motivation for being 'seen and heard';
tries to catch the attention and interest of others to show himself or herself off;
shows individuality and competes noticeably with others to claim the social scene.

c) Adaptation-ready. The child:
- is able to contribute to the execution of activities in the group thanks to his or her great attention to the intentions of others and good social 'ear';
- is seldom a soloist;
- is able to follow others' proposals and agenda–through social acts, not in the form of passive submission;
- only marks his or her intentions weakly and to a modest extent;
- is able to follow an agenda determined by others–but has minimal influence on the group's agendas; he or she seldom opposes other children's agendas;
- often experiences that his or her proposals are ignored by others who are more dominant and better at applying various instruments of power–often he or she experiences talking without anyone paying attention;
- often leaves it up to others, adults, and children, to choose his or her social contacts, others making contact to other children on his or her behalf.

d) Socially isolated behaviour. The child:
- generally has only sporadic interactions with others;
- receives few and weak initiations of contact from other children. As a consequence, the child is often ignored or overlooked by others;
- uses more active strategies to avoid or break a social contact;
- experiences lack of success in making contact with others, and this results in minor attention to the other children's intentions as well as in reduced ability to follow these intentions;
- withdraws from interactions with other children and withdraws to inner fantasy world;
- sometimes may turn into a socially excluded child, if the isolation is severe and consistent.

Blind children often have difficulty in becoming or showing socially competent in interactions on their own with sighted friends. They may use self-marking behaviour as a necessity in order to be acknowledged–heard and seen–by the others. However, positive self-marking behaviour may often develop into negative behaviour, because self-marking behaviour is only positive if it is adopted with moderation. Blind children's behaviour patterns may have some points of similarity with behaviour patterns that are normally observed in adaptation-ready and socially isolated children (Ingsholt, 2009). It is important to note that these differences in social skills affect the play behaviour. Many studies have shown that children with visual impairments show a high variability in social competence skills, a compromised social interaction and show that this limits the play behaviour: in kindergarten they are less enterprising, while only seldom they look for interactions with peers and propose games and activities (Celeste, 2006; Parsons, 1986; Skellenger et al., 1997; Zanandrea, 1998).

In addition, Schneekloth (1989) discovered that blind children spent playing alone 56% of their play time, while low-vision children spent only 33% of this time alone, compared to 14% in children without any visual impairment. The same author also found out that sighted children spent most of their play time interacting with their peers, while visually impaired spent 1/3 of their play time in interactions with adults.

A comprehensive study of Fraiberg (1977) compared visually impaired and sighted children in their play activities. She discovered that blind students had significant delays in many play areas–for example, they did not perform imitative play before 30-36 month. An earlier research of Fraiberg and Adelson (1973) suggested that even the concept of self in blind and low-vision children was delayed because of their poor and rare engagement in symbolic, pretend, and fantasy plays. According to the authors this is due to the fact that sighted children started to imitate the household life by taking care of a doll, for instance, at the age of 24 months, while blind children did not demonstrate this type of play before the age of 36-42 months.

Later, a similar study was carried by Troster and Brambring (1994). The authors concluded that sighted children engaged in more complex levels of play at an earlier age than the blind children did; the blind children interacted less frequently with their peers than the sighted children did; furthermore, the blind children preferred tactile-auditory games and toys and rarely engaged in symbolic games.

Similarly, other studies (Parsons, 1986; Lewis et al., 2000; Tioli, 2006) confirm a substantial difference in the playing capabilities of blind children, indicating that the blind child has a delay in the onset of mental image that later gives rise to the emergence of symbolic play. The blind child remains engaged for long in play activities that include: exploration of own body, and undifferentiated manipulation of an object, in a nonfunctional modality, without specific purposes. These are, therefore, activities of repetitive and stereotyped solitary play. Not only the symbolic play appears much later than in sighted children, that is in a span of time between the second year of life and the end of preschool age, but also the constructive play–where child learns to place objects in relation to each other (for example, to build a tower with toy blocks or doing a puzzle)–is compromised due to manual and bimanual coordination difficulties, less coordination and orientation abilities.

In 1995, the Bielefeld longitudinal study on early intervention and family counselling for blind infants and preschoolers (Brambring et al., 1995) assessed all areas of development, comparing the blind and sighted children's performances. In 2005, Brambring presented some results of the longitudinal studies held in the University of Bielefeld, which included the findings on 107 skills analysed in a comparative way between blind and sighted children, divided into four areas.

- Manual and daily living skills
- Gross motor skills
- Social interaction
- Language

Table 7.1. shows a few examples, where blind children experience serious delays in different play activities.

Table 7.1. Play delays in blind children (Brambring, 2005)

Skill	Sighted children (age in months)	Blind children (age in months)
Building a tower with three toy blocks	15	29
Finding two identical objects in a set of five objects	26	42
Beating a drum rhythmically with two drumsticks	11	37

One very comprehensive literature review on play in visually impaired children was made by Rettig (1994). One of the findings in this research was that vision and communication were both very important, especially in the case of social play with peers, and in this regard, some forms of play may be difficult to perform by blind or low-vision children. Furthermore, Rettig (cit.) adds that visually impaired children have limited play experience in their play, and these are due to delays in different developmental areas. This applies to a great extend to:

1. Practice play
2. Pretend or symbolic play
3. Social play
4. Play with rules
5. Creative play
6. Associative play

Visually impaired children demonstrate a delay in their symbolic play–at the age of 25,9 months (Rogers & Puchalski, 1984). Fariberg (1977) even prolonged this delay, stating that blind children do not participate in pretend and imitation play before 30-36 months of age. Fraiberg and Adelson (1973) suggested that the delayed acquisition of the concept of self in visually impaired children is associated with the delay in their symbolic play.

This point of view is confirmed more recently by Brambing (2004) who described the difficulty of the process of separation-individuation not only as a cause of limited self-perception of the child with visual impairment, but also as the cause of his or her late speech development, especially in regard to the late appearance of the first person singular. This last–that is the initial delay in language development–is also explained (Rowland, 1984; Hatwell, 2003) in relation to the lack of the prelinguistic child/mother dialogue through facial expressions and proxemics.

Brambing (2004) also underlined that, when symbolic play appears in the blind child, it is not based on the use of objects, rather on role-play games. This may be due to the fact that for the blind child it is easier to understand and use the process of symbolisation through acknowledging a similarity of reciprocal body movements and exchanges between people than through a similitude of objects. This hypothesis confirms that during the development of these children the emphasis is on the verbal aspects of their life, and also demonstrates that the initial language delay can be perfectly compensated.

On the other hand, some forms of play may not be so difficult for children with visual impairments, and they may feel engaged in them without great effort; as to the possible kinds of play activities, it is the case of, for example: functional play, constructive play play with language fantastic play, storytelling.

7.2 Strategies for Compensation of the Delays and Difficulties in Play by Children with Visual Impairments

Rettig and Salm (1992) suggested five strategies for intervention in order to support and to improve the play behaviours of young children with visual impairments:

1. Specific instructions for developing play skills
2. Use of toys
3. Adaptation of the environment
4. Including peers without disabilities
5. The role of adults

The first strategy includes actions as: a) providing the blind babies and infants with as many real objects as possible; b) helping symbolic play; c) avoiding the stereotyped behaviours and mannerisms and so on; d) enhancing sense of self to foster social development (Rettig, 1994); e) encouraging intrinsic motivation, active engagement, flexibility, spontaneity (Recchia, 1997).

The second strategy includes: a) demonstrating the child on how to use the different toys he or she has at home; b) providing the blind child more tactile and/or musical toys.

The third strategy suggests to help the visually impaired children to orient and move effectively and autonomously in their play environment and to feel comfortable and safe there. Schneekloth (1989) states that play environments that are appropriately designed for children with visual impairments need to be “accessible, safe, exciting and complex” (1989: 201). This strategy also includes to design ordinary learning environments opportunities for play and to adapt learning environments to make them accessible to the impaired child in inclusive contexts (Rogow, 1983; Staccioli, 2010).

The fourth strategy proposed to introduce gradually sighted playing companions to the visually impaired child (at first only one). In addition, Rettig and Salm (1992) suggested to provide some adult supervision when visually impaired and sighted children play together in order to encourage any spontaneous interactions and to avoid any discriminative behaviours. The interaction between the blind child and his or her peers is important not only for access to *associative* and *cooperative* play in view of his or her development and pleasure, but mostly to give them the opportunity to fully exercise one of their rights: in fact, participation in recreational, play, leisure, and sport activities, including those in the school system, is precisely cited in the UN Convention on the Rights of Persons with Disabilities (2006, Art. 31), historically most denied in case of sensory disability.

Lastly, the fifth strategy suggests different levels of participation of adults (parents, early carers, and other professionals) in the visually impaired child’s play. Rettig (1994) refers a gradual withdrawal of parents and other adults from playing with the children with visual impairments. Tioli (2006) also advances that the role of the adult becomes more and more insignificant during these children’s development. On the contrary, the play of these children should be first led by the adult, who should commensurate it to the child’s ability but also propose higher level of performance; not too high, however, so that the child does not feel frustrated and the attempt to increase the complexity of play does not fail. Only at that point, when the child has successfully experienced some types of play and feels more confident with this activity, a play free from adult intervention can be proposed.

7.3 Conclusion

Many authors underline the significance of play for the overall child development. Experiences from the early periods of child’s life, when play is the main activity a child is engaged in, form the basis for subsequent social development in adults (Sutton-Smith, 2001; Ingsholt, 2009; Tzvetkova, 1994). Augusto Romagnoli was one the first educators to indicate that the blind child acquires through play the awareness of self, of others. and of their otherness, experiences solidarity and cooperation. So, play must be pursued as a principle of maximum socialisation (Romagnoli, 1924).

However, visually impaired children are able to build their play skills similarly to sighted children, with some difficulties or delays. As the Russian educator and psychologist Vygotskij noted: “In the end there is no fundamental difference between the sighted and the blind child [...] and the whole process of development is one and the same for blind and sighted children” (1983:95).

References

Alliegro, M. (1993). *L’educazione motoria dei minorati della vista. Il gioco e lo sport* [Motor education of persons with visual impairments. Play and sport]. Roma, I: Armando.

Bateman, B. (1963). *Reading and Psycholinguistic Processes of Partially Seeing Children*. Arlington, VA: Council for exceptional children.

Brambring, M., Beelmann, A., Buitenhuis, S., Hecker, W. Kurp, C., Licher-Eversmann, G., & Muellerm A. (1995). Fruefoerderung blinder Kinder. *Konzepzion und Peadogogische Psychologie*, 37(4), 173-183.

Brambring, M. (2004). *Lo sviluppo nei bambini non vedenti. Osservazione e intervento precoce* [Visually impaired children’s development. Observation and early intervention]. Milano, I: Franco Angeli.

Brambring, M. (2005, August). *Assessing Developmental Differences in Blind versus Sighted Children*. Keynote speech at the ICEVI European conference, Chemnitz, G. Retrieved from: http://www.icevi-europe.org/chemnitz2005/icevi-chemnitz2005.pdf.

Celeste, M. (2006). Play Behaviours and Social Interactions of a Child Who Is Blind: In Theory and Practice. *Journal of Visual Impairment & Blindness*, 100(2), 75-90.

Erwin, E. J. (1993). Social participation of young children with visual impairments in specialized and integrated environments. *Journal of Visual Impairment & Blindness*, 8(7), 138-142.

Fraiberg, S. (1977). *Insights from the Blind. Comparative Studies of Blind and Sighted Infants*. New York, NY: New American Library.

Fraiberg, S., & Adelson, E. (1973). Self-representation in language and play: Observations of blind children. *Psychoanalytic Quarterly*, 42, 539-562.

Garvey, C. (1990). *Play*. Cambridge, MA: Harvard University Press.

Gomulicki, B. R. (1961). *The Development of Perception and Learning in Blind Children*. Cambridge, UK: Cambridge University: The psychological laboratory (mimeo).

Hayhoe, S. (2014, June). *A Grounded Theory Investigation into the Philosophical and Pedagogical Theories of Play by Bind and Visually Impaired Children*. Presented at the 6th Biennial Conference of the International Froebel Society “Play, Self-activity, Representation and Development”, Canterbury, UK.

Hatwell, Y. (2003). *Psychologie cognitive de la cécité précoce* [Cognitive psychology of early blindness]. Paris, F: Dunod.

Ingsholt, A. (2009, July). *Social Inclusion of 4-6-years-old Blind Children. What Social Competencies Do Blind Children Need? How Can They Best Be Strengthened*? Presented at the ICEVI European conference, Dublin, Ireland.

Kirk, S., & Gallaghar, J. (1979). *Educating exceptional Children*, Boston, MA: Houghten Mifflin Company.

Lewis, V., & Collis, G. M. (1997). *Blindness and Psychological Development in Young Children*. Leicester, UK: British Psychological Society.

Lewis, V., Norgate, S., Collis, G., & Reynolds, R. (2000). The consequences of visual impairment for children's symbolic and functional play. *British Journal of Developmental Psychology*, 18(3), 449-464.

Litvak, A, G. (1985). Тифлопсихология. [Psychology of the Blind]. Moscow, RUS: Education.

Lowenfeld, B. (1948). Effects of Blindness on the Cognitive Functions of Children. In: B. Lowenfeld (Ed), *Berthold Lowenfeld on Blindness and Blind People. Selected Papers* (pp. 67-78). New York, NY: AFB.

MacCuspie, P. A. (1992). The social acceptance and interaction of visually impaired children in integrated settings. In: S. Z. Sacks, L. S. Kekelis, & R. J. Gaylord-Ross (Eds.), *The Development of Social Skills by Blind and Visually Impaired Students: Exploratory Studies and Strategies* (pp. 83-102). New York, NY: American Foundation for the Blind.

Parsons, S. (1986). Function of play in low vision children: I. A review of the research and literature. *Journal of Visual Impairment & Blindness*, 80(3), 627-639.

Parsons, S. (1986). Function of play in low vision children: II. Emerging patterns of behavior. *Journal of Visual Impairment & Blindness*, 88(6), 777-784.

Recchia, S. L. (1997). Play and Concept Development in Infants and Young Children with Severe Visual Impairments: A Constructivist View. *Journal of Visual Impairment & Blindness*, 91(4), 401-416.

Rettig, M. (1994). The play of young children with visual impairments: characteristics and interventions. *Journal of Visual Impairment and Blindness*, 88(5), 410-420.

Rettig, M., & Salm, K. (1992, April). *The Importance of Play in the Early Childhood Special Education Curriculum*. Paper presented at the 70th Annual Conference of the Council for Exceptional Children, Baltimore, Maryland.

Rogers, S. J., & Puchalski, C. B. (1984). Development of Symbolic Play in Visually Impaired Young Children. *Topics in Early Childhood Special Education*, 3(4), 57-63.

Rogow, S.M. (1983). Social routines and language play: Developing communication responses in developmentally delayed blind children. *Journal of Visual Impairment & Blindness*, 77(1), 1-4.

Romagnoli, A. (1924). *Ragazzi ciechi* [Blind children]. Bologna, I: Zanichelli.

Rowland, C. (1984). Preverbal communication of blind infants and their mothers. *Journal of Visual Impairments and Blindness*, 78(7), 297-302.

Rowland, W. P. (1985). *Being Blind In The World*. Pretoria: South African National Council for the Blind.

Sacks, S. K., Kekelis, L. S., & Gaylord-Ross, R. J. (1992). *The Development of Social Skills by Blind and Visually Impaired Students: Exploratory Studies and Strategies*. New York, NY: American Foundation for the Blind.

Sandler, A-M, & Wills, D.M. (1974). Preliminary notes on play and mastery in the blind child. *Journal of Child Psychology*, 1(3), 7-19.

Schneekloth, L. H. (1989). Play environments for visually impaired children. *Journal of Visual Impairment & Blindness*, 83, 196-201.

Skellenger, A., & Hill, E. (1994). Effects of a shared teacher-child play intervention on the play skills of three young children who are blind. *Journal of Visual Impairment & Blindness*, 88, 433-445.

Skellenger, A. C., Rosenblum, L. P., & Jager, B. K. (1997). Behaviors of Preschoolers with Visual Impairments in Indoor Play Settings. *Journal of Visual Impairment & Blindness*, 91(6), 519-530.

Sommer, D. (2003). Barndomspsykologiske facetter. Århus, DK: Systime A/S.

Staccioli, G. (2010). Includere nel gioco. In: S. Besio (Ed.), *Gioco e giocattoli per il bambino con disabilità motoria* [Play and toys for the child with motor impairment] (pp. 73-81). Milano, I: Unicopli.

Sutton-Smith, B. (2001). *The Ambiguity of Play*. Cambridge and London: Harvard University Press.

Tioli, E. (2006). Dallo spazio aptico alla rappresentazione immaginativo-motoria [From the haptic space to the imaginative-motor representation]. *Tiflologia per l'integrazione*, 6, 4-16.

Troster, H., & Brambring, M. (1994). The play-behavior and play materials of blind and sighted infants and preschoolers. *Journal of Visual Impairment and Blindness*, 88(5), 421-432.

Tzvetkova, M. (1994). Играта при зрително затруднените деца. [Play in Visually Impaired Children]. Preschool Education, 7(8), 48-50.

Vygotskij, L.S. (1983). Собрание сочинений, том пятый: **Основы Дефектологии.** [Collected Works, Volume Five: Fundamentals of Defectology]. Moscow, RUS: Education.

Wills, D. M. (1968). Problems of play and mastery in the blind child. *British Journal of Medical Psychology*, 41, 213-222.

Zanandrea, M. (1998). Play, social interaction and motor development: practical activities for preschoolers with visual impairments. *Journal of Visual Impairments and Blindness*, 92(3), 176-188.

Natalia Amelina and Vardit Kindler

8 Play in Children with Communication Disorders

All mental processes during the childhood – perception, memory, attention, imagination, thinking, purposeful behaviour – develop through direct engagement with language.

Connected with consciousness in general, human language joins various relationships with all mental processes. Being a mediated system of signs, language reconstructs all mental processes of the person, reaching the level of volitional, conscious functioning. It is clear that language and thinking are closely connected with each other.

Clinical, medical, psychological, and pedagogical research, as well knowledge in the professional fields of language, show that children with communication disorders face specific challenges associated with mental processes: attention, perception, memory, thinking (Hughes, 2010).

Not only the development of cognition suffers from the presence of communication disorders, but, as it is immediately evident, the area of social development is affected by the restriction of possibilities to exchange comments, ideas, proposals with their peers that these children unavoidably experience. This fact has, in turn, consequences on the overall child development, and in particular, on the language development itself. Solutions should be found as soon as possible to substitute and/or to support the communication of these children, exactly to the purpose of avoiding secondary acquired limitations.

However, before characterising the play skills of these children, it is important to identify the term 'communication disorders'. Most of the existing studies identify children with communication disorders as a heterogeneous group characterised by a range of difficulties in speech and language.

Communication disorders due to language difficulties are often associated with other kinds of disabilities, such as intellectual and physical impairments or autism spectrum disorders;[1] or, they can be present as the only or prevalent neurological disorder, as in the case of dysphasia.

Language disorders are usually diagnosed by using tests of nonverbal intelligence (Guralnick et al., 2003; Catts et al., 2002; Kelly & Sally, 1999). Other diagnosis instruments aimed at evaluating the detailed characteristics of the impairment can be used to study single levels, including those of phonology, morphosyntax, semantics, pragmatics, and discourse (Leonard, 1998; Tager-Flusberg & Cooper, 1999; Tallal & Benasich, 2002).

1 Further deepening is contained in the related chapters of this book.

8.1 Some Characteristics of Mental Processes in Children with Communication Disorders

Psychological research states that limitations in communication often result in difficulties in some intellectual activities, such as to analyse purposefully the conditions of an intellectual task, or to find its essential elements and to single out the right correlations among them; to make comparisons; to generalise; to make abstractions; and to implement control over intellectual activities. The main obstacle for these children is the difficulty to plan their activities (and play is among them) as a logical series of consecutive specific actions. At the same time, the performance of separate operations usually does not cause difficulties to them.

The most critical limitation in the intellectual activity of these children is the insufficient development of separate operations, while the whole plan of the activity is comprehended and carried out by the child (Usanova, 1995). Lurija (1998) noted that communication disorders result in cross-functional social and developmental limitations.

All types of limitations in language and speech development, according to various authors, decrease the volume of information that can be acquired by a child; furthermore, the accuracy of the acquired information decreases and the processing of language development slows down. In general, they have negative effects on a child's play.

Children with speech impairments due to visible damages to the effector apparatus – for example, in the case of lip and/or palate cleft malformations[2] – often meet difficulties in interacting with their peers and experience emotional stress.

Stuttering[3] in childhood is often related to the limitation of attention concentration; according to some authors, they often show impulsivity that leads them to try to reach a goal in a hurry, without the needed concentration. Also, in this case, their relationships with peers can be restricted due to a reluctance induced by their awareness of their verbal expression difficulties; they look shy and sometimes isolated, do not trust their own abilities, are reluctant to take a central role in play and prefer to observe or to adopt supporting roles.

Children with dysarthria[4] have severe difficulties or limitations in developing effective attention abilities (both sustaining and shifting) as their peers; they may find it difficult to understand language and may need additional explanation or prompts

2 Cleft lip and palate malformations, also known as oro-facial cleft, is a group of congenital impairment, that includes cleft lip and/or cleft palate.

3 Stuttering is a speech disorder in which the flow of speech is disrupted by involuntary repetitions and prolongations of sounds, syllables, words, or phrases as well as involuntary silent pauses or blocks in which the person is unable to produce sounds.

4 Dysarthria is a motor-speech disorder resulting from neurological injury of the motor component of the motor-speech system.

when they are given verbal tasks or instructions. They also may show difficulties in switching from one task to another, as well as a little interest in the results of the performed activity.

According to Ippolitova and Mastyukova (1985), children with dysarthria might find logical thinking challenging. Sometimes, they are not used to make connections between subjects and phenomena of the world around – similarities and distinctions – on the basis of usual and expected cues; for example, the classification of subjects is carried out on the basis of the concrete situational environments of their communication, while they find it difficult to make generalisations.

Developmental dysphasia,[5] which is a total restriction in speech related to language disorders, can radically influence the child's social and psychological development; it interrupts and affects the most important means and ways of communication, thus causing a slow down of the cognitive development. Children with developmental dysphasia may experience a slow rate in the information reception and in the quality of language processing, which, in turn, also worsens the communication abilities: for example, they may find it difficult to analyse tasks, make comparisons, generalise, make abstractions. Attention stability and switching attention can be also difficult. All these problems might cause them face possible emotional and psychological challenges, such as irritability, emotional instability, lack of initiative, and so on. A constant support to their motivation can be useful for their involvement.

8.2 Play Activities of Children with Communication Disorders

Psychological research states that preschool children with speech and language disorders, in comparison with their non-impaired peers, linger long in the manipulation of objects expected in the stage of practice play; in addition, role-playing games are mastered by them much more slowly, with quite repetitive and elementary contents. If the child starts playing with his/her peers, he or she quickly 'slides off' the role assigned to him or her, thereby breaking the rules. This could be a reason for these children often are excluded from play with their peers or they are given only supporting roles in the play activities.

The negative factors influencing the play of children with communication impairments are related to the fact that their language is considered poor by their peers, or that their play companions do not correctly understand what they are saying, due to their imperfect pronunciation of language or the adoption of unusual morphosyntactic structures.

5 Developmental dysphasia is a severe impairment of the language system that is considered a result of cortical speech zones defect appearing in the preverbal period.

All these limitations may cause difficulties mainly to the symbolic play, where the use of language is almost imperative, for pretending an object is something else and agreeing on this fact with other children, for building up – alone or in group – play situations, with roles, conversations, events, and so on, or even for using the language as the core itself of play, for example, in narrations, in language jokes.

A number of researchers have, in fact, investigated the relationships between language disorders and difficulties in symbolic play (Lewis et al., 2000; Lyytinen et al., 2001; McCune, 1995; Watt et al., 2006). Many authors, for instance, noted that children with communication disorders face difficulties in handling peer conflict (Hart et al., 2004; Horowitz et al., 2007); they are seldom capable of behaving in an assertive way, get frustrated easily, and are more dependent on adults for assistance than other children (McCabe & Marshall, 2006; Picone & McCabe, 2005). For all of the aforementioned reasons, they are less likely than the typically developing child to engage in cooperative make-believe play.

Preschool children with severe speech and language disorders often tend to play with toys silently, in a solitary way; only sometimes, they may accompany their own actions with sounds or emotional exclamations. While communicating with peers, they tend to replace words with deictic words or gestures, or sometimes with single words. The most frequent emotional aspect of the relationship of a child with a toy is displayed in the form of exclamations, sounds, single words, onomatopoeias.

In the case that these children show also difficulties in understanding the language and the situations in which they are, the core essence of the play and mainly the game rules remain inaccessible for a long time; they tend to repeat their actions and to imitate what has been already done in other similar situations.

Another type of play that is really compromised in the case of communication disorders is the game with rules: in fact, in this case, not only the rules should be deeply understood – and they are mainly shared verbally in the children's group – but they should then be adopted, sometimes with the need of negotiating with the peers their right application.

All the play situations, within any type of play, in which a space is necessarily devoted to negotiation, mediation, to presenting and explaining one's own reasons and ideas about the play development, can be challenging for these children. They can, of course, take part in games and in collective play activities, but they rely mostly on imitation and repetition, while as soon as the need for a dialogue is foreseen, they would need support; otherwise, they will soon abandon the play activity itself.

8.3 Environmental Factors: Augmentative Alternative Communication

A number of researches noted that the differences in the play activities between children with communication disorders and the other children can be strongly related to environmental factors and that the impairments can be widely reduced with the right environmental supports, strategies, and tools.

The quality and quantity of interactions with peers, the adult's ability to respond to the child's communication efforts, the accessibility of play areas for those facing additional impairments (e.g., children with motor and/or visual impairments), and the availability of adapted toys or assistive technologies for play and communication are the factors that influence the child's participation in play and leisure activities.

Due to its focus on participation, the adoption of Augmentative and Alternative Communication (AAC) strategies is a variable influencing the child's engagement in play and his or her participation in social interactions with peers.

According to ISAAC, AAC is "a set of tools and strategies that an individual uses to solve everyday communicative challenges".[6] AAC is an umbrella term that encompasses the communication methods used to supplement or replace speech for persons who experience impairments in the production or comprehension of spoken or written language.

AAC is based on devoted intervention approaches (Glennen, 2000) that combine the child's natural communication abilities (including any existing speech or vocalisations, gestures, manual signs, facial expressions) with aided forms of communication, including the use of communication boards with symbols[7] (pictures, photographs, line drawings, symbols, printed words) or the use of speech-output communication devices.

AAC is a multimodal approach, permitting a child to use a wide range of modes to communicate messages and ideas. As communication abilities may change over time, although sometimes very slowly, the choice of the AAC system or code at one age is not to be considered definitive, and it may be modified as a child grows and develops (Beukelman & Mirenda, 2005).

The roles an AAC system plays will vary depending on an individual child's needs; they can augment the existing natural speech, provide a primary output mode for communication, provide an input and an output mode for language and communication, and serve as a language intervention strategy (Light & Drager, 2007).

If a child needs an AAC communication system, it is very important that it is used during all his or her daily activities, to express his or her desires and ideas, to comment about what happens. Of course, in these cases, the AAC system as well as its low- or high-tech supports should be available in his or her contexts of life above all to support the daily activities, first of all for playing. The most common and well-known

6 ISAAC is the International Society for Augmentative and Alternative Communication; www.isaac-online.org.

7 The symbols and pictograms that are used can be created on purpose, on the basis of the single child's needs, or belong to internationally established codes, as in the case of PIC, PCS, Blissymbolics, and so on.

role of the devices is to provide an output mode for communication. Technological devices, in particular, offer children with communication impairments the access to "the magic and the power of communication" (Light & Drager, 2007). It is also of utmost importance, in fact, that the child is offered appropriate AAC systems as early as possible, so that the communication mode becomes a substantial aspect of his or her life. Thanks to the use of AAC, the child can grow, learn, develop under the social and cognitive respect.

But, to reach these objectives, the related technological devices should respond to some particular characteristics (Light & Drager, 2002): among the others, they should be 'appealing, capturing'; they must be easily integrated into all aspects of daily living; they might 'provide access to the magical power of communication'; they should grow with children as they develop. The design of these tools is, thus, extremely important (Light et al., 2004), possibly as similar as possible in its main features to the children's first toys, above all as they should be used in collective spaces, where other children also live and play; they must be attractive also to the peers of children with communication impairments, and become a usual and well-known mean for communication and for playing together.

As it has been argued, the type of play that is mostly influenced by a communication impairment is the symbolic play. By providing the impaired child the right symbols he or she needs to fully participate, AAC can prove very useful to support – without underestimating the evidence from practice that in some cases play should be explicitly taught (Barton & Wolery, 2008) – all the symbolic play activities, from the pretend play to the use of dolls and other toys able to create environments and make-believe situations, or even role-playing.

AAC can, of course, also be adopted to tell stories, by substituting the written text that usually accompanies the children's book stories with symbols, and this option gives a group of children the possibility to share the same activity; if they are very young, symbols can be as the unique text, without the alphabetical one.

Furthermore, the possibility to manage a communication code gives the child with communication impairments the opportunity to play different roles within the group and also within the family: for example, he or she can tell a joke, pretend that an object is a different one, give instructions to other persons – peers or adults – on how they should act, or respond, and on the roles they should assume; if the device has also a voice output, the child might also take part in nursery rhymes, can even sing with the others.

If the communication impairment is not accompanied by other types of impairments, the child should not experience difficulties in constructive play; thanks to the AAC, he or she can be anyway supported in following the different steps of a complex activity, such as building a home for puppets, using Lego bricks, cooking biscuits, and so on, and this is much more true if a physical impairment is associated and the child has severe limitations in fine movements.

As to the games with rules, AAC can be used as a support to explain the rules to the child with communication impairments, in case this is needed, but it can also be concretely used as a tool for mediating relationship with peers – for example, to indicate the alternate turn, to score points, to interrupt the game if needed and makes one's arguments heard.

This short review can illustrate clearly that AAC is a very powerful tool for making it possible and improving the play of children with communication impairments; as it is easy to understand, communication being the most important way to be in contact with the world around, these play activities should be patently supported to enhance and empower their potential inclusive aspects. As soon as communication is available, it is also possible to build up new worlds – real or invented – and to modify them, to share ideas and projects, to discuss, to impose one's own points of view, to claim victory, or to admit defeat.

This not only favours but implies that inclusive contexts are offered to these children, so that they can fully benefit of the related opportunities for communicating, and for playing; on the other hand, the greater validity of the inclusive model has been confirmed in the field research (Foreman, Arthur-Kelly & Pascoe, 2004): students using AAC in general classrooms were involved in significantly higher levels and more frequent communicative interaction than their peers in special classrooms.

8.4 Conclusion

The topic of play of children with communicational disorders has not been studied in-depth until now and even the existing studies give only some suggestions about the reasons that are at the basis of the differences existing in their play activities. Too often, it has been assumed that children with communication disorders have inherent limitations in play when, sometimes, differences in play skills might be explained more easily by environmental variables.

However, it is important to take into consideration the possible reasons of play differences, cited by a certain number of the aforementioned researches.

- The cognitive activities of children with communication disorders are impacted by difficulties in their attention, in particular, the attention focus, the ability to switch, the attention stability, and so on.
- There are difficulties in memory – acoustic, visual, verbal, and logical. These limitations have an impact on the other mental processes, such as perception, thinking, self-organisation of purposeful activity, and they make speech even more difficult.
- Speech and language disorders limit the social contacts and communication of these children with their peers and/or with adults. This influences in a negative way the development of the cognitive processes, and in turn, changes also the nature of their play.

It is very important for adults to understand the verbal and nonverbal signals while playing with the child. The aforementioned strategies and assistive technologies can play a significant role of support to parents and educators.

References

Barton, E. E., & Wolery, M. (2008). Teaching Pretend Play to Children With Disabilities. A Review of the Literature. *Topics in Early Childhood Special Education*, 28(2), 109-125.

Beukelman, D., & Mirenda, P. (2005). *Augmentative and alternative communication: Management of severe communication impairments (4th ed.).* Baltimore, MD: Paul H. Brookes Publishing.

Catts, H. W., Fey, M. E., Tomblin, J. B., & Zhang, X. (2002). A longitudinal investigation of reading outcomes in children with language impairments. *Journal of Speech, Language, and Hearing Research*, 45, 1142–1157.

Foreman, P., Arthur-Kelly, M., & Pascoe, S. (2004). Evaluating the Educational Experiences of Students with Profound and Multiple Disabilities in Inclusive and Segregated Classroom Settings: An Australian Perspective. *Research and Practice for Persons with Severe Disabilities*, 29(3), 183-193.

Glennen, S. (2000, January). AAC assessment myths and realities. Paper presented at the *ASHA SID 12 Leadership Conference on Augmentative and Alternative Communication*, Sea Island, GA.

Guralnick, M. J., Hammond, M. A., & Connor, R. T. (2003). Subtypes of nonsocial play: Comparisons between young children with and without developmental delays. *American Journal on Mental Retardation*, 108, 347–362.

Hart, K., Fujiki, M., Brinton, B., & Hart, C.H. (2004). The relationship between social behavior and severity of language impairment. *Journal of Speech, Language, and Hearing Research*, 47, 647–662.

Horowitz, L., Westlund, K., & Ljungberg, T. (2007). Aggression and withdrawal related behavior within conflict management progression in preschool boys with language impairment. *Child Psychiatry and Human Development*, 38(3), 237-253.

Hughes, F. (2010). *Children, play, and development (4th edn)*. London, UK: Sage.

Kelly, D. P., & Sally, J. I. (1999). Disorders of speech and language. In M. D. Levine, W. B. Carey, & A. C. Crocker (Eds.), *Developmental–behavioral pediatrics (3rd edn)*, (pp. 621-631). Philadelphia: Saunders.

Leonard, L. B. (1998). *Children with specific language impairment*. Cambridge, MA: MIT Press.

Lewis, V., Boucher, J., Lupton, L., & Watson, S. (2000). Relationships between symbolic play, functional play, verbal and non-verbal ability in young children. *International Journal of Language and Communication Disorders*, 35, 117-127.

Light, J. C., & Drager, K. (2007). AAC technologies for young children with complex communication needs: State of the science and future directions. *Augmentative and Alternative Communication*, 23(1), 204-216.

Light, J. C., & Drager, K (2002). Improving the Design of Augmentative and Alternative Technologies for Young Children. *Journal of Assistive Technology*, 14(1), 17-32.

Light, J. C., Drager, K, & Nemser, G. J. (2004). Enhancing the Appeal of AAC Technologies for Young Children: Lessons from the Toy Manufacturers. *Journal of Assistive Technology*, 20(3), 137-149.

Lurija, A. R. (1998). Язык и сознание [Language and conscious]. Rostov-na-Donu, RUS: Fenix.

Lyytinen, P., Poikkeus, A. M., Laakso, M. L., Eklund, K., & Lyytinen, H. (2001). Language development and symbolic play in children with and without familial risk of dyslexia. *Journal of Speech, Language and Hearing Research*, 44, 873-885.

Mastyukova E. M., & Ippolitova, M. V. (1985). Нарушение речи у детей с церебральным параличом [Speech disorders in children with cerebral palsy]. Moscow, RUS: Education.

McCabe, P. C., & Marshall, D. J. (2006). Measuring the social competence of preschool children with specific language impairment: Correspondence among ratings and behavior observation. *Topics in Early Childhood Special Education*, 26(4), 234-246.

McCune, L. (1995). A normative study of representational play at the transition to language. *Developmental Psychology,* 31(2), 198-206.

Picone, M., & McCabe, P. C. (2005). The reliability and discriminant validity of the Social Interactive Coding System with language impaired preschoolers. *Journal of Early Childhood and Infant Psychology*, 1, 113-128.

Tager-Flusberg, H., & Cooper, J. (1999). Present and future possibilities for defining a phenotype for specific language impairment. *Journal of Speech, Language, and Hearing Research*, 42, 1275–1278.

Tallal, P., & Benasich, A. A. (2002). Developmental language learning impairments. *Development and Psychopathology*, 14, 559–579.

Usanova, O. N. (1995). Дети с проблемами психического развития Издательство [Children with problems of psychological development]. Moscow, RUS: NPC Korrektsiya.

Watt, N., Wetherby, A., & Shumway, S. (2006). Prelinguistic predictors of language outcome at three years of age. *Journal of Speech, Language, and Hearing Research*, 49, 1224-1237.

Serenella Besio and Natalia Amelina

9 Play in Children with Physical Impairment

9.1 Motricity and Mind

According to numerous researchers (Sechenov, 1952; Pavlov, 1937; Oliverio, 2007), motor actions play an important role in the formation of mind; they affect learning and are at the basis of language development. In fact, movements, motor schemes, and physical relationships with the real world can cause a development in mental logic, underpin logical construct, and are at the basis of the understanding of the cause/effect relationships and of the chaining of sequences of thoughts.

Between motricity and mind, there is a complex interrelation, which could be described as cyclic: a movement can exert some consequence on the surrounding environment, and due to the perception of these consequences, new, modified movements can be produced; this relationship appears very clearly in a newborn (Barbeau, 1990). According to this approach, it is not the movement that satisfies the mind's needs, while it is the mind that performs the actions (Oliverio, 2007). Some authors recently sustain that motor control resides in nervous system, body, and environments "viewed as dynamical systems in continuous interaction" (Turvey, 2009:3).

The ontogeny seems to reproduce in this sense the phylogeny: some neurophysiologists (Calvin, 1990) sustain, in fact, that the evolution of some motor behaviours caused, historically, the creation of a 'motor logic' based on subsequent steps, and this provoked—from the motor and the premotor cortex areas—a sort of contamination towards the Broca area of language, to 'inspire' the generation of sequences of syllables.

For Lurija (1973), the human brain is a sort of archive of complex motor schemes—that he defined 'kinetic melodies' to refer to their fluidity and availability in different moments of daily life. The techniques of brain imaging have then greatly contributed to the knowledge of such schemes. The major achievement in these last decades is the discovery of the role of the mirror neurons (Gallese et al., 1996) located in the premotor areas: it has been demonstrated, in fact, that there is a parallelism between the brain areas fired while acting a movement and in imagining it or viewing it performed by another or even by a robot. Studies concerning these relationships are currently done in the neuroscience field, within the framework of the so-called 'embodied cognition' (Wilson, 2002), and even if final conclusions have not been reached, the undergoing experimentations about the relationships between some areas of cognition (language, memory, visual perception, and so on) and the movement, obtain various results, they always demonstrate interesting clues of secure interconnection (Tomasino & Rumiati, 2013; Tomasino et al., 2011).

The child's motricity depends on a complex mixture of predispositions and experiences, on the brain's capability to record the motor actions perceived by sight, and on the progressive acquisition of motor actions that are corrected and refined through trials and errors; they are finally stored in a memory able to code them as schemes and to make them available in a fluid and stereotyped form (Oliverio, cit.).

9.2 Children with Physical Impairments

As a consequence of what is discussed in the previous paragraph, it is possible that a delay in the development of motor skills, or the presence of various degrees of motor impairments, may have an adverse impact on the mental and cognitive development of the child.

A physical impairment—both congenital and acquired—creates substantial limitations to physical ability or motor skills; when it is related to a problem of the central nervous system—as in the case of cerebral palsy (CP),[1] ataxia, traumatic brain injury—it may be accompanied, at different degrees, by intellectual and neuropsychological impairments,[2] language and speech disorders, sensory disabilities, as well as emotional and social difficulties (Tingle, 1990). It could also be related to a damage to the peripheral nervous system and/or to the effector organs (muscles, joints, and bones); the functional situation of these children is often severe—as in the case of some types of muscular dystrophy, and of spinal muscular atrophy— with rapid worsening; and also when it is less dramatic—as in the case of juvenile rheumatoid arthritis—it limits the movement possibilities of the children, thus restricting their ability and also their willingness to be active and to participate.

In many cases, motor impairments can prevent the child from acting in an autonomous way in his or her daily activities, and in its turn, these limitations cause insufficient development of his or her sensory and perception capabilities, as well as low self-esteem and self-efficacy.

Very often, these children need the adoption of various assistive devices and supports for movement and for communication. Of course, this implies a special organisation of their daily life, because they need to be trained to the use of these tools for long periods, and in turn, this may create restrictions in social participation as well as difficulties at the psychological level, mainly with respect to self-construction and self-representation.

1 Cerebral Palsy affects 2% of the newborns in technologically advanced countries.

2 Some Italian researches have highlighted the high presence (the two-third) of an intellectual disability in children with CP with a mean lower performance of one standard deviation (Cioni et al., 1993).

In the case of CP, the possible association of intellectual and sensorial impairments,[3] as well as the possible absence or severe impairment of speech,[4] may cause a very complicated overall functioning of these children and may make challenging to support and to empower their play abilities.

Speech disorders may disadvantage their communication with peers, as it might be difficult to understand them, or an alternative communication system should be adopted. These aspects, together with the possible difficulties to the emotional sphere reported in the clinic literature,[5] can result in social participation restriction, if appropriate inclusive contexts are not established.

The most recent interpretative model of CP highlights the spontaneous adaptive effort of the affected children, by considering the symptoms as the result of this effort, within a complex situation of functional and biological systems that are intertwined but superordinate to the performance. Thus, the motor component is no more the only variable to consider, but it should be analysed together with the others: perceptive, attentional, motivational, cognitive, and emotional-affective. All these components tend to reach the best possible balance, while facing the inner and outer needs of the child; in infancy, play is without a doubt the ideal bridge between the external world and the internal world of the child (Voltolin & Obino, 2011).

But, play is also a matter of social inclusion: within the framework offered by the International Classification of Functioning (WHO, 2001), many studies—conducted to single out the possible correlations between the physical impairment and the level of participation of children (Wright et al., 2008)—concluded that they are at risk of reduced participation, interpreted both as a subjective and an objective experience (Law et al., 2006). A comprehensive literature analysis found that they "experience greater participation restriction than their peers without impairment and the participation of children with CP or other neurological impairments was more restricted than that of other disability groups" (Imms et al., 2008:363). Furthermore, activities are more passive, mainly organised at home and lack variety (Shikako et al., 2008). Other surveys (Majnemer et al., 2008; Orlin et al., 2010; Palisano et al., 2011) sustain that the intensity of participation is influenced by some determinants of the child and his or her family: higher participation is related to higher gross motor function, higher enjoyment, younger age, and higher family orientation; moreover,

3 According to the clinical literature, slowness of the thought processes and inertness of thinking are typical of children with CP. Insufficiency of the highest cortical functions can also be shown in a delayed development of the representations of space and time, of the processes of phonemic analysis, and synthesis and problems of astereognosis (Mastyukova & Ippolitova, 1985).

4 Speech development of children with CP is characterised by disorders on many components: lexical, grammatical, and phonetic or phonemic. Most frequently, they suffer from dysarthria or even anarthria.

5 Emotional excitability or irritability, sometimes mental block, disinhibition. In some cases, low motivation to activity and aspiration to restricted social contacts are referred.

social supports and environmental services also play an important role in increasing the degree of participation. Denmark, with its welfare system, has been singled out as one of the European countries where participation is best sustained (Michelsen et al., 2008); another direct correlation has been found with the type of school system, even if in Italy—a country that can boast a 'totally inclusive' system—the level of participation is not so satisfying for families.

9.3 Technologies and Children with Physical Impairments

The severity of the physical impairment of these children has been often considered a scientific challenge to create solutions for supporting both their activities and participation; more than in the case of children with other types of impairments, technologies can become a significant part of their life, and their use as tools for rehabilitation is highly represented in the field literature. In particular, the play of children with physical impairment has been investigated: for this reason, in what follows, a short presentation of the area in more general way is necessary to review, in the next paragraphs, the existing literature with respect to the characteristics of the various types of play.

A particular role can be played by Assistive Technologies (ATs)[6] whose name should not remind the idea of being passively 'assisted' rather the construct of 'supports for independence': in fact, they are mainly addressed to support the autonomy of the impaired persons, to let them reach their goals, and to decrease the workload of assistants. Many AT products[7] have been developed, classified at international level according to their scope,[8] and made available to the users according to national regulations.

Also, mainstream technologies are often used as tools for rehabilitation, enjoyment, and leisure time. Due to the extraordinary and rapid changes in the technological field, it is quite natural to think that they could offer these children what they need, provide experiences they might not do by themselves, and consequently, improve the perception of their own capabilities, thus enhancing their self-efficacy (Bandura, 1977). This has been the case, for example, of some proposals to use the virtual reality (VR) environments (Reid & Campbell, 2006), which can provide these

6 "Any product or technology-based service that enables people of all ages with activity limitations in their daily life, education, work or leisure" (AAATE, 2003; www.aaate.net). Other definitions have been established by international bodies, such as ISO 9999.

7 WHO prefers the expression *Assistive Health Products* to underline their importance to support the person's health condition, that is, a status of complete well-being: physical, psychological, and social: http://www.who.int/phi/implementation/assistive_technology/gate_full_final_report_july_2014.pdf.

8 The Standard ISO 9999:2011 classifies the assistive products for persons with disabilities according to their function in three hierarchical levels: www.iso.org/obp/ui/#iso:std:iso:9999:ed-5:v1:en.

children a sense of mastery and self-efficacy. In effect, VR has proved to provoke fun in children with physical impairment, also when it is used for rehabilitation purposes (Bryanton et al., 2006).

Nowadays, AT and mainstream technology are often used together to create original systems called ‘assistive solutions’,[9] which can also assemble environmental modifications and even some personal assistance. They are highly personalised, as the solution found for one individual is usually different from the one that proved useful for another individual (Andrich, 2013). In addition, the same AT products are not useful to the same degree for different persons, and they can play different functions according to the users’ needs; a single piece of technology cannot solve a situation, rather it should be adapted to the type and context of use (Besio, 2007). For all these reasons, the process of choice of AT should be managed by a multi-professional team with the active participation of the child and also of his or her parents during the decision phase.

Another important field in which technology is fast developing and experimenting is robotics. Play has been adopted as a promising testing area:[10] “the underlying assumption is that providing tailored means to encourage play through a robotic toy will break down barriers for development through play, fostering individual development up to the persons full potential” (Kronreif, 2009:222). These researches also intend to envisage a ‘new potential role for advanced robotics in society’, seen as a possible contributor to enhance the following three aspects: quality of life, social inclusion, learning, and therapy. A very promising area of development of this field is the use of robots to reveal cognitive skills of children with disabilities, which is particularly difficult in case of severe impairments (Cook et al., 2010).

Any AT—including robotic tools—that supports the motor actions of the child “may enable development” (Cook & Polgar, 2008:67). Unfortunately, finding the suitable assistive solution for children with severe physical impairment could be difficult and challenging for them, and they should be supported and motivated to gain the desired result: their major involvement can be, obtained, again, by recurring to technologies that can be able to playfully engage them in the training activities (Adams et al., 2013).

Bringing together a very broad discussion, we can say that products, technologies in general, and AT solutions, which are all included within the ICF domain of Environmental Factors, can become powerful facilitators—if correctly identified and

---

9 See also the ‘Position Paper’ of AAATE, 2012. http://aaate.net/wp-content/uploads/sites/12/2016/02/ATServiceDelivery_PositionPaper.pdf.

10 Anyway, the application of robotics to disability, and in particular to physically impaired children is mainly addressed to rehabilitation; experimentation results are frequently assessed with respect to rehabilitation objectives, even when they are used for engaging and ludic activities (Rahman et al., 2015).

situated in a person's daily life—for the activity of a person with disability and his or her social participation. In the case of the child with a physical impairment, they are used as a support for typical activities of the age, including play; they can, in fact, offer occasions to experiment, to grow, to have fun, to become autonomous, to increase participation and social inclusion.

But, products and technologies can also pose to be barriers for play: this could happen in the case of toys and playgrounds that are not usable or accessible to the child with physical impairment, for example, if they are not easy to grasp, to be explored, manipulated, used.

The need to develop effective technologies to support these children's play has become a meaningful objective of the scholars in the field, while abilities to assess and improve the usability and the accessibility of play tools, technologies, and contexts are still to be implemented and widely disseminated.

9.4 Play and Children with Physical Impairments

The scientific interest towards the play activities of children with motor and/or physical impairments has increased during the last 20 years. Playfulness has been found significantly lower in children with CP than in typically developing ones (Okimoto et al., 2000): in particular, their 'play age' is referred to their mental abilities and not to their chronological age. Something similar was reported by Harkness and Bundy (2001): their experimentation resulted in scores of 'exuberance' higher in children with physical impairment—but without any intellectual impairment—than in typically developing ones.

The presence of an intellectual impairment and its complex interrelation with the physical impairment seems to be extremely relevant data; in particular, it can determine the capacities, the possibilities, and the preferences of the motor-impaired child when playing. Dallas et al. (1993a) found that children with CP showed a deficit of assertiveness during play, while Brodin (1999) stresses passivity, lack of attention, and concentration.

Howard (1996) hypothesised a possible correlation between these behavioural data and the living habits of these children, often obliged to reduce drastically leisure time and fun, due to the intense and frequent rhythms of physical rehabilitation.

The lack of initiative not only seems to be a consequence, but also a cause of a reduction of the play occasions. This is true, for example, for physically impaired children who show a significant delay in speech development and a consequent reduction of communicative competence, or who depend on others for their movement. In such cases, their social interactions decrease, and as a consequence, they acquire a reduction in play initiative and in peer relationships (Harper & McCluskey, 2002).

The most recent research results put specific emphasis on the role of the environmental competence and proposals; a wide inter-individual variety exists among children, and child neurologists stress that differences should not always considered pathological: it is important to observe, interpret, and exploit the child's adaptive capabilities, or, as Brazelton says, the 'best performance' within the limitation (Bottos, 2003). As some severely impaired children can express their will and ability to act and participate, any prognosis should be made with caution, taking advantage of their desires as well as of the environmental proposals; and this is true also—or mainly—for what concerns play (Mortenson & Harris, 2006).

Certainly, adaptability and modifiability can occur only within an environment that is competent to welcome, interpret, and support the child's needs and proposals of interaction. On the one hand, the environment should be correctly structured and oriented towards the cognitive development (Bronfenbrenner, 1975), and on the other hand, the children's activities should be facilitated, for example, by choosing the right toys, which can be usable and contemporarily can offer the right level of challenge to stimulate their motivation, their fun, and finally, their development (Brodin, 2005).

In what follows, the main aspects that the different types play reveal in the case of children with physical impairment will be presented.

9.4.1 Practice Play

Through exploratory activities, the child becomes able to make inferences on the surrounding reality, to integrate perceptive and motor schemes in a sort of elementary interpretation of the world. The child with physical impairment is particularly disadvantaged in such activities: the inferential processes seem to proceed from the motor abilities, and particularly, from their use within the play activities.

In fact, there are physically impaired children who due to their functional limitations cannot reach, manipulate, use the objects and are only onlookers of their peers' play activities; some of them do not know the special condition of tension and density that can be related to play because they do not perceive themselves as the owners of their own thoughts, or they cannot understand the rules, the peers' proposals and suggestions.

Bruner (1968) sustained that the concrete motor act is not decisive to determine the child's development, while it is important the intention to make it, the capability to formulate a hypothesis, and to plan the activity; this reflection could be interesting to explain why in some cases children with severe motor impairment can show typically developing intellectual abilities. But, this interpretation should not lead to underestimate the possible consequences—for the child's development—of a reduced motor activity and particularly of a lack of practice play. To elicit play abilities, to favour curiosity, and to increase relationships of the young motor-impaired children, some solutions have been experimented (Butler, 1986) in trying to give them as much mobility as possible, as early as possible; this brought to the development of some robotic vehicles for children, such as PALMIBER (Ceres et al., 2005; Raya et al.,

2013). These projects are based precisely on the need to offer these children proper opportunities to explore and interact with space, 3D objects, and people around them (Cook & Polgar, 2008). Therefore, to drive these vehicles, children should be able to carry out purposeful actions, to interact with objects and use them as tools; to make this possible for children with physical impairment, who cannot manipulate objects directly, on-purpose adaptations and assistive solution systems have been implemented, including switches or other devices (Cook et al., 2000). Verburg (1987) found a decrease in parents' protectiveness while the child is able to demonstrate more confidence in mobility.

Another productive line of research and intervention is conducted in a less-strict technological area, and it is aimed to increase awareness of teachers and professionals in the field and to improve their knowledge and competence in assessing and choosing products, toys, and technologies for the play of children with physical impairment: in fact, these objects must be suitable for their functional needs and their further development.

9.4.2 Symbolic Play

As already noted, in some children, especially in the case of CP, severe physical impairment is accompanied by a deep impairment in language and/or speech acquisition and use. The development of effective and competent symbolic functions is also related to the integrity of the gross and fine motor functions: this means, the ability to use objects for pretend play, but also to use language to create and 'inhabit' invented worlds. Anyway, some findings in literature (Martinoni & Scascighini, 1997) describe cases of symbolic play in the absence of a completely developed speech capability, mostly if strategies of alternative communication have been established.

If some researches indicate significant differences in play abilities between children without and with developmental language difficulties, being lower in this last case (Casby, 1997), other ones demonstrate that pretend play does not show a stable correlation with the use of verbal language (Lyytinen, 1991) even if language seems to have a pulling role for the development of the symbolic function as a whole.

Other studies underline the strong influence exerted on symbolic play by the child's socio-economical context and by the parents' educational styles (Bornstein et al., 1996).

Symbolic play can be greatly compromised in the case of children with physical impairment due to motor difficulties—think, for example, to play with dolls that should be manipulated in a fine manner; very often the play companion helps the child in overcoming these difficulties "becoming the child's hand" (Brizzolara et al., 2005).

The developmental leap for this type of play is the ability to deal symbolically with objects, and ATs can be of great help if they are designed accordingly to these children's possible needs: play activities can now be organised along sequential steps—like within a narration—and, in case that their speech skills are poor, the symbols of augmentative codes should be implemented on their toys and play objects. Research demonstrates that the adoption of the suitable ATs to support symbolic play can enable learning and associated development.

An interesting high-tech perspective in this sense is the 'social robotics', which creates a direct interaction between the user and the robot; an example of this type is IROMEC,[11] which was tailored towards becoming a social mediator, to foster social and cooperative play. More than having 'symbolic' features in itself, IROMEC has been used as a mediator for building up symbolic play activities (thus also overcoming some limits it demonstrated about its attractiveness as an enjoyable tool), as it happened during experimentations: "Between the first and the last session, the adults try to enhance the play situation. They try to enrich it, to build more stimuli and ideas to make children's attention more focused on the activity; in terms of play theory, it could be said that they try to enhance the play scenarios available on the IROMEC, that mainly belong to the sensorimotor level, by translating them to a symbolic and imaginative level" (Besio et al., 2013:147).

9.4.3 Constructive Play

It was Smilansky who first stressed the need to separate, in the child's development, the acquisition of gestures from their use for doing things, creating, constructing. This idea opened the possibility of separating the practice from the constructive play, which includes in fact the growing child's abilities of planning and realising ideas that are in his or her mind and very quickly mingle with the newly acquired symbolic abilities, in a developmental spiral of incremental complexity (Smilansky & Shefatya, 1990).

Smilansky's approach is particularly productive and rich in new ideas for studying the play of children with physical impairments because it has facilitated the raising of research projects in the field of engineering and robotics. One interesting example of this is given by the robot system Play ROB, designed as an assistive system to help severely impaired children in playing with Lego bricks; in this case, the robot is not the toy, but it helps to use the toy (Kronreif et al., 2005).

Some authors suggest that, for the cognitive development of children with motor impairment, it is not essential to be able to act on the objects of the world around them, rather to be able to make inferences on it and to represent these actions in their minds. Anyway, this assertion has been somehow questioned by some case studies

---

11 It is the acronym of *Interactive Robotic Social Mediators as Companions*, IST-FP6-045356, Specific Targeted Research or Innovation Project.

that used educational and robotic technologies (Besio, 2004; Kronreif et al., 2005). They put into evidence, in fact, a not complete effectiveness of these representational mechanisms, as children, when asked to act concretely on objects according to precise plans, showed weaknesses in planning exactly their actions and in verifying the obtained results, as well as in correcting the actions that were wrong according what they had in mind.

More recently, some contexts of ‘constructive play’ with commercial robots have been used to study the cognitive skills of children with disabilities (Cook et al., 2010); the detailed analyses of the subsequent so-called ‘micro-behaviours’ needed to manage and control a robot within a constructive play activity as well as the categorisation of the increasing cognitive skills implied by these play activities are the basis to build up a theoretical framework for relating robot skills with child-developing cognitive skills. This result will be unavoidable in the future to foster new knowledge and develop new tools in the field.

Starting from this point, for example, the use of Lego Mindstorms robots as ATs for giving children with physical disabilities the possibility to play through manipulation has been tested for the purpose of measuring the possible effects on playfulness (Rincon et al., 2013a); robots were used for play at home with the intention of supporting free play of a child with CP. The results demonstrated that playfulness increased with the introduction of a robotic intervention, and, even more interesting, this happened thanks to the creation of play scenarios in which robots became the mediator of symbolic activities with dolls, blankets, and ‘scenes’ to represent. The results related to the previous study indicate that the child’s communicative utterances increased as well as the mother’s responsiveness to the child’s initiative (Rios et al., 2013b); this was interpreted as a consequence of a major engagement and motivation in play of both.

9.4.4 Play with Rules

Children with physical impairments can approach this type of play in many cases by recurring to the use of an IT tool; if the accessibility issue is correctly solved and the suitable game is chosen in relation to their cognitive abilities, it is possible to offer them a virtual environment that is adaptable and usable.

These kind of games have been already experimented successfully (Weiss et al., 2003; Reid, 2004): for example, adolescents with CP showed appreciation and enjoyment in using these tools, in strict correlation with the cognitive workload requested by the game.

Reid and Campbell (2006) reported a successful use by children with CP (with non-disabled peers) of a VR environment—managed by a video camera as a device for capturing and tracking—for playing games of volleyball and snowboarding. They perceived VR as an 'equaliser' of abilities with their peers, and this fostered feelings of competence and acceptance by the others.

One of the main problems of mainstream videogames for these children is their requirement of playing fast and being action-oriented. Hernandez et al. (2013) created a specially designed videogame—called 'exergame'—to avoid the need for time-sensitive actions and to keep the game pace slow, which have been tested with children with CP, both to achieve the right physical activity and fun.

9.5 Social Aspects of Play in Children with Physical Impairments

Since decades, we know that the mere exposition to toys is not sufficient either to increase the number of play activities or to adopt new types of play, while the adult's mediation reveals much more importance in this respect, to model the child's play behaviour.

But, in case of children with disabilities, there is a risk that parents adopt a 'diagnostic' attitude (Brodin, 2005),[12] focussed on recovery and rehabilitation of the impairment, rather than on 'unproductive' activities such as play, which is considered a 'wasted time'. The same author proposes that parents should be trained to adopt specific abilities, such as withstanding the slowness of gesture execution of their children and their delayed comprehension of play situations, as well as acquiring the needed competence to liven concentration on the task and to maintain it for long time.

In some studies of the field, children with physical impairments have been described as frustrated by their motor impairment and poorly trust in themselves as players and play companions (Pollock et al., 1997); they have been also described as snivelling and emotionally unstable, not very friendly (Sprinkle & Hammond, 1997). Spencer-Cavaliere and Watkinson (2010) sustain that they feel 'included' in a physical activity when they gain entry to play, feel like a legitimate participant, have friends. According to Skär (2002), they improve their own perception if they use ATs that can give them more autonomy in play activities, without recurring to the aid of an adult.

On the other hand, their limitation on activity and restriction in participation causes a huge decrease in their possibility to make choices and may even produce loss of awareness on their right to have control on their own lives; this is an important loss because it is exactly the possibility to influence one's own environment and to interact with people that makes it possible to reduce the feeling of helplessness (Weiss et al., 2003).

But, the real and most important infant social learning happens during play activities with peers. Children with disabilities, mainly those with severe impairments

12 Not all the studies are in the same frame (Malone & Landers, 2001; Lane & Mistrett, 1996).

such as CP, tend, regardless of the chronological age, to adopt subaltern roles in the group (Dallas et al., 1993a, 1993b); play dyads are, for this reason, more fruitful if the impaired child is the youngest one, thus benefiting by control behaviours adopted by the other (McGillicuddy-De Lisi, 1993).

Cooperative behaviours in siblings (one of them with CP) increase in time as well as pro-social and care behaviours; time probably increases the awareness about the reciprocal needs and supports in building a good relationship: the non-disabled sibling becomes more and more competent in interpreting the sister or brother's wishes and in complying with them, maintaining attitudes of support and physical proximity. This also results in increasing the impaired child's participation and attention to the play activities.

Therefore, children with CP find it difficult to start an interaction with their siblings, and this causes less probabilities to be involved in play activities and a major probability that the siblings take the control over the situation (Dallas et al., 1993a).

Specific characteristics related to the impairment can greatly influence the acquisition of play competences. The linguistic abilities play a primary role: children with good verbal competences are more likely to be involved in the peers' play activities (Stoneman et al., 1989; Harper & McCluskey, 2002); also, the cognitive competences influence the associative and collaborative types of play, because sometimes these activities prove to be too complex for an impaired child. Furthermore, children who are not autonomous in their movements and need some support for moving tend to rely on adults for entering the peers' group.

An Italian research some years ago (Catullo, 1984) verified that children with motor impairment but without any associated cognitive impairment were more popular among their peers, unless children who showed behavioural problems and difficulties to understand the rules or to comply with them, who were often left out. In addition, only 6% of the drawings of peers depicting children with motor impairments put into evidence signs of their impairments, for example, their technical aids. This fact was interpreted as a positive demonstration that these children are not seen as 'lacking' something, no child seemed interested in the 'disabling' aspects. The same experimental model has been reproduced in Italy (Besio, 2011), but different results were found. In fact, it was confirmed that only 8% of the children depicted wheelchairs or other technical aids of their peers, but these drawings were found in classes where the inclusive process was well established and effective, in which impaired children with disabilities obtained high preference scores in sociograms. This result seems to lean towards the opposite conclusion of the previous experiment: more precisely, it is possible that a positive experience and relationship with an impaired peer can contribute to improve general attitudes towards disability in general and to the perception of technical aids and other possible 'strange objects' as simply normal in the school context, as if they belonged to the whole inclusive community.

This conclusion could be interpreted within a line of studies, which identifies a direct correlation between the attitudes towards ATs and disability in general: negative attitudes towards disability (seen as weakness and dependence) are associated to a negative perception of AT (McMillen & Söderberg, 2002; Bender Pape et al., 2002), while in the meantime, positive attitudes towards disability also include a positive conception of technologies that are considered as tools that make it possible or favour the autonomy of a person.

References

Adams, K., Rios Rincòn, A. M., Encarnação, P., Piedade, G., Helmbold, B., & Tuck, C. (2013). Learning Switch Scanning Skills for Playing with Robots. In: P. Encarnação, L. Azevedo, G. J. Gelderblom, A. Newell, & N. E. Mathiassen (Eds.), *Assistive Technology: From Research to Practice* (pp. 360-365). Amsterdam, DK: IOS Press.

Andrich, R. (2013). Service Delivery Systems for Assistive Technology in Europe: A Position Paper. In: P. Encarnação, L. Azevedo, G. J. Gelderblom, A. Newell, & N. E. Mathiassen (Eds.), *Assistive Technology: From Research to Practice* (pp. 247-253). Amsterdam, DK: IOS Press.

Bandura, A. (1997). *Self-efficacy: The Exercise of Control.* New York, NY: WH Freeman & Co.

Barbeau, M. (1990). Processus interactifs mnésiques et comportamentaux après coma post-traumatique chez l'enfant [Mnestic interactive process and behaviours after post-traumatic coma of the child]. *Approche Neuropsychologique des Apprentissages chez l'Enfant*, 2, 20-22.

Bender Pape, T. L., Kim. J., & Weiner, B. (2002). The Shaping of Individual Meanings Assigned to Assistive Technology: A Review of Personal Factors. *Disability & Rehabilitation*, 24, 5-20.

Besio, S. (2011). *Gioco e giocattoli per il bambino con disabilità motoria* [Play and toys for the child with motor impairment]. Milano, I: Unicopli.

Besio, S. (2007). *Analysis of Critical Factors involved in using interactive robots for education and therapy of children with disabilities.* Deliverable 5.1. European Project IROMEC (Interactive RObotic MEdiators as Companions (IST-FP6-045356). Bruxelles: IROMEC Consortium. Retrieved from: www.iromec.org.

Besio, S. (2004). Using Assistive Technologies to Facilitate Play by Children with Motor Impairments: A Methodological Proposal. *Technology and Disability*, 16(3), 119-130.

Besio, S., Carnesecchi M., & Converti, R. M. (2013). *Prompt-fading Strategies in Robot Mediated Play Sessions.* In: P. Encarnação, L. Azevedo, G. J. Gelderblom, A. Newell, & N. E. Mathiassen (Eds.), *Assistive Technology: From Research to Practice* (pp. 143-148). Amsterdam, DK: IOS Press.

Bornstein, M. H., Haynes, O. M., Watson O'Reilly, A., & Painter, K. M. (1996). Solitary and collaborative pretense play in early childhood: sources of individual variation in the development of representational competence. *Child Development*, 67, 2910-2929.

Bottos, M. (2003). *Paralisi cerebrale infantile. Dalla "guarigione" all'autonomia. Diagnosi e proposte riabilitative* [Cerebral palsy. From healing to autonomy. Diagnosis and rehabilitation proposals]. Padova, I: Piccin.

Brizzolara, D., Brovedani, P., & Ferretti, G. (2005). Valutazione cognitiva e neuropsicologica [Cognitive and neuropsychological evaluation]. In: A. Ferrari, & G. Cioni (Eds.), *Le forme spastiche della paralisi cerebrale infantile. Guida all'esplorazione delle funzioni adattive* (pp. 183-216). Milano, I: Springer Verlag Italia.

Bryanton, C., Bossé, J., Brien, M., McLean, J., McCormick, A., & Sveistrup, H. (2006). Feasibility, Motivation, and Selective Motor Control: Virtual Reality Compared to Conventional Home exercise in Children with Cerebral Palsy. *CyberPsychology & Behavior*, 9(2), 123-128.

Brodin, J. (1999). Play in children with severe multiple disabilities: play with toys—a review. *International Journal of Disability, Development and Education*, 46(1), 25-34.
Brodin, J. (2005). Diversity of aspects on play in children with profound multiple disabilities. *Early Child Development and Care*, 175(7-8), 635-646.
Bronfenbrenner, U. (1975). Is early intervention effective? Some studies of early education in familiar and extra familiar settings. London, UK: Oxford University Press.
Bruner, J. (1968). *Processes of Cognitive Growth: Infancy*. Worcester, MA: Clark University Press and Barre.
Bundy, A. C. (1997). *ToP—The Test of Playfulness*. Fort Collins, CO: Colorado State University.
Bundy, A. C. (1999). *TOES—Test of Environmental Supportiveness*. Fort Collins, CO: Colorado State University.
Butler, C. (1986). Effects of Powered Mobility on Self-Initiated Behaviors of Very Young Children with Locomotor Disability. *Developmental Medicine & Child Neurology*, 28, 325-332.
Calvin, W. H. (1990). *The Cerebral Symphony*. New York, NY: Bantam.
Casby, M. W. (1997). Symbolic play of children with language impairment. A critical review. *Journal of Speech, Language and Hearing Research*, 40, 480-492.
Catullo, D. (1984). Come i bambini percepiscono l'handicappato fisico [How children perceive the physical impairment]. *Psicologia Italiana*, 6(1), 16-20.
Ceres, R., Pons, J. L., Llanarys, C., & Azevedo, L. (2005). A robot vehicle for disabled children. *IEEE Engineering in Medicine ad Biology Magazine*, 24(6), 55-63.
Cioni, G., Paolicelli, P. B., Sordi, C., & Vinter, A. (1993). Sensorimotor development in cerebral palsied infants assessed with the Uzgiris-Hunt Scales. *Developmental Medicine and Child Neurology*, 35, 1055-1066.
Cook, A., Encarnação, P., & Adams, K. (2010). Robots: Assistive technologies for play, learning and cognitive development. *Technology and Disability*, 22, 127-145.
Cook, A. M., & Polgar, J. M. (2008). *Cook & Hussey's Assistive Technologies: Principles and Practice*. St. Louis, MO: Mosby.
Cook, A., Howery, K., Gu, J., & Meng, M. (2000). Robot enhanced interaction and learning for children with profound physical disabilities. *Technology and Disability*, 13(1), 1-8.
Dallas, E., Stevenson, J., & McGurk, H. (1993a). Cerebral-palsied children's interactions with siblings. I. Influence of severity of disability, age and birth order. *Journal of Child Psychology and Psychiatry*, 34(5), 621-647.
Dallas, E., Stevenson, J., & McGurk, H. (1993b). Cerebral-palsied children's interactions with siblings. II: Interactional structure. *Journal of Child Psychology and Psychiatry*, 34(5), 649-671.
Gallese, V., Fadiga, L., Fogassi, L., & Rizzolatti, G. (1996). Action Recognition in the Premotor Cortex. *Brain*, 119(2), 593-609.
Harkness, L., & Bundy, A.C. (2001). The Test of Playfulness and children with physical disabilities. *The Occupational Therapy Journal of Research*, 21, 73-89.
Harper, L. V., & McCluskey, K. S. (2002). Caregiver and peer responses to children with language and motor disabilities in inclusive preschool programs. *Early Childhood Research Quarterly*, 17, 148-166.
Hernandez, H. A., Zi Ye, T. C., Graham, N., Fehlings, G., & Switzer, L. (2013). Designing Action-based exergames for Children with Cerebral Palsy. In: S. Bødker, S. Brewster, P. Baudisch, M. Beaudouin-Lafon, & W. E. Mackay (Eds.), *Proceedings of the SIGCHI 2013 Conference on Human Factors in Computing Systems* (pp. 1261-1270). New York, NY: Association for Computer Machinery.
Howard, L. (1996). A comparison of leisure-time activities between able-bodied children and children with physical disabilities. *The British Journal of Occupational Therapy*, 59(12), 570-574.
Imms, C., Reilly, S., & Dodd, K. (2008). Diversity of Participation in Children with Cerebral Palsy. *Developmental Medicine & Child Neurology*. 50, 363-369.

Kronreif, K. (2009). Robot Systems for Play in Education and Therapy of Disabled Children. In: I. R. Rudas, J. Fodor, & J. Kacpzyk (Eds.), *Towards Intelligent Engineering and Information Technology* (pp. 220-234). Berlin-Heidelberg, D: Springer.

Kronreif, G., Prazak, B., Mina, S., Kornfeld, M., Meindl, M., & Fürst, M. (2005). PlayRob. Robot-Assisted Playing for Children with Severe Physical Disabilities. *Proceedings of ICORR 2005, 9th International Conference on Rehabilitation Robotics*. Chicago, IL.

Lane, S. J., & Mistrett, S. G. (1996). Play and assistive technology issues for infants and young children with disabilities: A preliminary examination. *Focus on Autism and Other Developmental Disabilities*, 11(2), 96-104.

Law, M., King, G., King, S., Kertoy, M., Hurley, P., Rosenbaum, P., ... & Hanna, S. (2006). Patterns of Participation in Recreational and Leisure Activities among Children with Complex Physical Disabilities. *Developmental Medicine & Child Neurology*, 48, 337-342.

Lyytinen, P. (1991). Developmental trends in children's pretend play. *Child care, health and development*, 17, 9-25.

Lurija, A. R. (1973). *The Working Brain. An Introduction to Neuropsychology*. New York, NY: Basic Books.

Majnemer, A., Shevell, M., Law, M., Birnbaum, R., Chilingarayan, G., Rosenbaum, P., & Poulin, C. (2008). Participation and enjoyment of leisure activities in school-aged children with cerebral palsy. *Developmental Medicine & Child Neurology*, 50, 751-758.

Malone, M.D., & Landers, M.A. (2001). Mothers' perceptions of the toy play of preschoolers with intellectual disabilities. *International Journal of Disability, Development and Education*, 48(1), 91-102.

Martinoni, M., & Scascighini, G. (1997). *Pedagogia specializzata e informatica. Esperienze e realizzazioni in Ticino* [Specialized and computerized pedagogy. Experiences and realization in Ticino]. Lucerna, CH: SZH/SPC.

Mastyukova, E. M., & Ippolitova M. V. (1985). *Speech Impairments of Children with Cerebral Palsy*. Moscow, RUS: Prosvesheniye.

McGillicuddy-De Lisi, A. V. (1993). Sibling interactions and children's communicative competency, *Journal of Applied Developmental Psychology*, 14, 365-383.

McMillen, A. M., & Söderberg, S. (2002). Disabled Persons' Experience of Dependence on Assistive Devices. *Scandinavian Journal of Occupational Therapy*, 9(4), 176-183.

Michelsen, S. I., Flachs, E. M., Uldall, P., Eriksen E. L., McManus, V., Parkes, J., ... & Dickinson, H. O. (2009). Frequency of Participation of 8-12-year-old Children with Cerebral Palsy: A Multi-centre Cross-sectional European Study. *European Journal of Paedriatic Neurology*, 13(2), 165-177.

Mortenson, P. A., & Harris, S. R. (2006). Playfulness in Children with Traumatic Brain Injury. A Preliminary Study. *Physical & Occupational Therapy in Pediatrics*, 26(1-2), 181-198.

Obino, L., & Voltolin, G. (2011). *Idee di gioco nella riabilitazione neuromotoria: una analisi critica*. In: S. Besio (Ed.), *Gioco e giocattoli per il bambino con disabilità motoria* [Play and toys for the child with motor impairment] (pp. 17-27). Milano, I: Unicopli.

Okimoto, A. M., Bundy, A., & Hanzlik, J. (2000). Playfulness in children with and without disability: Measurement and intervention. *American Journal of Occupational Therapy*, 54, 73-82.

Oliverio, A. (2007, January). *The Acting Mind. The role of motricity in mental representation processes*. Montessori Centenary Conference, 1907-2007, Rome, I. Retrieved from: www.oliverio.it/ao/didattica/Montessori%20English.htm.

Orlin, M., Palisano, R. J., Chiarello, L. A., Kang, L.-J., Polanski, M., Almasri, N., & Maggs, J. (2010). Participation in Home, extracurricular, and Community Activities among Children and Young People with Cerebral Palsy. *Developmental Medicine & Child Neurology*, 52, 160-166.

Palisano, R. J., Chiarello, L. A., Orlin, M., Oeffinger, D., Polansky, M., Maggs, J., Bagley, A., & Gorton, G. (2011). Determinants of Intensity of Participation in Leisure and Recreational Activities by Children with Cerebral Palsy. *Developmental Medicine & Child Neurology*, 53(2), 142-149.

Pavlov, I. P. (1937). *Lections on Big Brain Hemisphere Work.* Leningrad, RUS: OGIZ.
Pollock, N., Stewart, D., Law, M. Sahagian-Whalen, S., Harvey, S., & Toal, C. (1997). The meaning of play for young people with physical disabilities. *The Canadian Journal of Occupational Therapy*, 64(1), 25-31.
Rahman, R. A., Hanapiah, F. A., Basri, H. H., Malik, N. A., & Yussof, H. (2015). Use of Humanoid Robot in Children with Cerebral Palsy: the Ups and Downs in Clinical experience. *Procedia Computer Science*, 76, 394-399.
Raya, R., Rocon, E., & Ceres, R. (2013). Robotic Vehicles for Assisted Mobility in Cerebral Palsy. In: J. L. Pons, D. Torricelli, M. Pajaro (Eds.), *Converging Clinical and Engineering Research on Neurorehabilitation* (pp. 1123-1127), Berlin-Heidelberg, D: Springer.
Reid, D. (2004). The influence of virtual reality on playfulness in children with cerebral palsy: A pilot study. *Occupational Therapy International*, 11(3), 131-144.
Reid, D., & Campbell, K. (2006). The Use of Virtual Reality with Children with Cerebral Palsy: A Pilot Randomized Trial. *Therapeutic Recreation Journal*, 40(4), 255-268.
Rios Rincon, A., Adams, K. D., Magill-Evans, J., & Cook, A. M. (2013a). Changes in Playfulness with a Robotic Intervention in a Child with Cerebral Palsy. In: P. Encarnação, L. Azevedo, G. J. Gelderblom, A. Newell, & N. E. Mathiassen (Eds.), *Assistive Technology: From Research to Practice* (pp. 161-166). Amsterdam, DK: IOS Press.
Rios Rincon, A., Sirard, K., Wainer, A., & Adams, K. (2013b). *LEGO Robot promoting mother-child communication during free play: A pilot study with a child with severe motor impairment.* Communication at the Rehabilitation Engineering and Assistive Technology Society of North America (RESNA) Annual Conference. Retrieved from: www.resna.org/sites/default/files/legacy/conference/proceedings/2013/PDF%20Versions/Computers%20and%20Communication/Rincon.pdf.
Sechenov, I. M. (1952). *Physiology and Psychology. Selecta. Volume 1.* Moscow, RUS: Academy of Sciences Publishing House.
Shikako-Thomas, K., Majnemer, A., Law, M., & Lach, L. (2008). Determinants of Participation in Leisure Activities in Children and Youth with Cerebral Palsy: Systematic Review. *Physical & Occupational Therapy in Pediatrics*, 28(2), 155-169.
Skär, L. R. N. (2002). Disabled children's perceptions of technical aids, assistance and peers in play situations. *Scandinavian Journal of Caring Sciences*, 16(1), 27-33.
Smilansky, S., & Shefatya, L. (1990). *Facilitating Play.* Silver Spring, MD: Psychological and Educational Publications.
Spencer-Cavaliere, N., & Watkinson, .J. (2010). Inclusion understood from the perspective of children with disability. *Adapted Physical Activity Quarterly*, 27(4), 275-293.
Sprinkle, J., & Hammond, J. (1997). Family, Health, and Developmental Background of Children with Developmental Coordination Disorders. *Australian Educational and Developmental Psychologist*, 14(1), 55-62.
Stoneman, Z., Brody, G. H., Davis, C. H., & Crapps, J. M. (1989). Role relations between children who are mentally retarded and their older siblings: Observations in three in-home contexts. *Research in Developmental Disabilities*, 10, 61-76.
Tingle, M. (2005). *The Motor Impaired Child.* Abingdon, UK: Taylor & Francis (1st ed. 1990).
Tomasino, B., & Rumiati, R. I. (2013). At the mercy of strategies: the role of motor representations in language understanding. *Frontiers in Psychology*, 4(27).
Tomasino, B., Skrap, M., & Rumiati, R. I. (2011). The role of the human motor hand area in mental rotation: Neuropsychological Evidence. *Journal of Cognitive Neuroscience*, 23, 2068-78.
Turvey, M. T. (2009). Nature of Motor Control: Not Strictly "Motor", not quite Control. In: D. Sternad (Ed.) *Progress in Motor Control. A Multidisciplinary Perspective, Advances in Experimental Medicine and Biology* (pp. 3-6; vol. 629).

Verburg, G. (1987). Predictors of successful powerful mobility control. In: K. M. Jaffe (Ed.), *Childhood powered mobility: developmental, technical and clinical perspectives.* Washington, D.C.: RESNA Press.

Weiss, P. L., Bialik, P., & Kizony R. (2003). Virtual reality provides leisure time opportunities for young adults with physical and intellectual disabilities. *Cyber Psychology and Behaviour*, 6(3), 335-342.

Wilson, M. (2002). Six Views of Embodied Cognition. *Psychonomic Bulletin & Review.* 9(4), 625-636.

World Health Organisation (2001). International Classification of Functioning Disability and Health. Geneva, CH: WHO.

Wright, F. V., Rosenbaum, P. L., Goldsmith, C. H., Law, M., & Fehlings D. L. (2008). How do Changes in Body Functions and Structures, Activity, and Participation Relate in Children with Cerebral Palsy? *Developmental Medicine & Child Neurology*, 50, 283-289.

Sylvie Ray-Kaeser, Evelyne Thommen, Laetitia Baggioni, and Miodrag Stanković

10 Play in Children with Autism Spectrum and Other Neurodevelopmental Disorders

Autism spectrum disorder (ASD) is a complex mental condition manifested by a wide range of cognitive, emotional, and neurobehavioural disabilities. ASD begins early in childhood (before the age of three) and lasts throughout life. Core deficits cause substantial impairments in social interaction and communication as well as the presence of fixed, stereotyped patterns of behaviour and a lack of interest in peers (APA, 2013). The first signs for the parents are that their child does not react to their presence nor responds to his or her name (despite the fact that hearing is intact) or is focusing on certain objects for a long time without initiating contact with people (Baron-Cohen, 2004). Moreover, a change of setting does not modify the core features of their behaviour, which differentiates ASD children from children with other developmental disorders (Stanković et al., 2012).

From this point of view, as a neurodevelopmental disorder, ASD shares many characteristics with those psychiatric conditions that typically manifest early in development. *Neurodevelopmental disorders* are "characterized by developmental deficits that produce impairments in personal, social, academic or occupational functioning" (DSM-5; APA 2013:31). They include disorders such as intellectual disability, specific learning disorders, communication disorders, attention-deficit hyperactivity disorder, and motor disorders. Comorbidity has long been recognised in children with neurodevelopmental disorders, which reflects some overlapping causes and underlying neurological abnormality (Kaplan et al., 1998).

10.1 Play Skills of Children with ASD and Other Neurodevelopmental Disorders

Multiple skills (cognitive, psychomotor, and relational) are required for playing, especially playing with peers (Perrin, 2011), and difficulties in playing are part of the core symptoms in ASD. Although many researchers describe the particularities of play amongst children with ASD, there are still misunderstandings and confusions about their actual ability to play. These children seem less playful than their peers, showing repetitive behaviours with objects, and restricted play interests (Benson et al., 2006). The way they play is characterised by certain fixations: they exhibit "preoccupations ranging from a fascination with objects to an intense focus on arcane topics" (Wolfberg et al., 2012:57).

The described behaviours may occur as a result of a range of varying overlapping difficulties. *Sensory integration dysfunctions* are frequently associated with ASD

(Rogers et al., 2003; Watling et al., 2001). Current estimates show that 45 to 96% of the children with ASD have difficulty in processing sensory stimuli (Ben-Sasson et al., 2009; Lane et al., 2010). A child's difficulty in processing and integrating sensory inputs affects participation in play activities (Schaaf & Mailloux, 2015). Over-sensitivity to noise, light, smell, or touch, also called sensory defensiveness (corresponding to a low threshold for response to stimuli), may manifest in play as avoidance of movement and restricted play preferences (Schaaf et al., 2011). On the contrary, sensory insensitivity or sensory seeking (high threshold) may manifest as reduced social interaction and difficulties in functioning or excessive movement and manipulative play in order to self-regulate the child's sensitivity level. Inattention may result from sensory-seeking behaviours, which makes the child switch from one activity to another, so that it interferes with play (Lane et al., 2010).

Children with ASD have been found to show similar motor difficulties as children with *developmental coordination disorders (DCD)* (Dewey et al., 2006; Green et al., 2009). Motor coordination difficulties, such as poor balance, eye-hand coordination, and decreased ability to plan and execute motor tasks, create social isolation and restrict participation in play (Cairney, 2015). Numerous researchers have highlighted the need to feel concerned about the consequences of impairment in motor coordination skills on children's playfulness and participation in physical play (Kennedy-Behr et al., 2013; Poulsen & Ziviani, 2004). Preschool children with coordination impairments show a lower developmental play age and engage less frequently in play than their typical peers (Kennedy-Behr et al., 2013). School-aged children with DCD avoid school playgrounds and engage less in physical and social play (Smyth & Anderson, 2000).

Children with ASD have *impaired joint attention, decreased imitation,* and *social imagination,* which are all skills necessary for symbolic play and pretend play (Jarrold, 2003). *Social interaction disturbance,* which is the core symptom in ASD, has very heavy consequences for social play (Nadel, 2002; Ten Eycke & Müller, 2015). Moreover, reduced social play of children with ASD has been linked to particularities in *cognitive and emotional development* (Jordan, 2003), while difficulties in *verbal and nonverbal communication* limit the capacity of children with ASD to engage in play with others (Wolfberg et al., 2012).

A *theory of mind impairment* is often discussed in ASD children to explain their difficulties in symbolic play (e.g., dolls, tea parties) or 'hide and seek play' that involves mental representations to imagine being another person or put oneself in a playing partner's shoes (Thommen et al., 2014). *Executive functions disorder* is also available as an explanatory theory of ASD functioning and the difficulties involved in planning series of actions to 'create' the play, be attentive, be able to change the rules of play, and even inhibit a response when they have to take turns (Thommen et al., 2014). However, due to the heterogeneity of the symptoms in ASD, it is important to avoid asserting simply that all children with ASD have the same difficulties in playing.

All these primary skills needed for a child with ASD to play have to be learnt. To do so, individual play may initially be prioritised before group play, which will later ensure the generalisation of learning. Social cognition may then become the main focus.

Different methods of *individual intervention* for children with ASD exist to develop the skills needed for play. Even though they need more structured play and external cues to develop their play skills (Tanta & Knox, 2015), the structural component of the environment might be problematic for them. When it is very controlled, as in the *Applied Behavioural Analysis* (ABA) method (Lovaas, 1987), it can lead to difficulties in the generalisation of learning (Wood et al., 2013). Other methods of intervention such as *Pivotal Response Training* (PRT) (Koegel & Kern Koegel, 2006), *Treatment and Education of Autistic and Communication Handicapped Children* (TEACCH) (Schopler, 1997), or *Early Start Denver Model* (ESDM) (Rogers & Dawson, 2010), use the most natural environment while being structured and encourage behaviour initiation in order to facilitate the generalisation of learning. These interventions are the most effective for developing play skills because they use the child's strengths and seek inner motivation through activity more than external rewards (Luckett et al., 2007). Using the specific skills of children with ASD to increase their motivation in play seems essential. Specific skills related to the characteristics of ASD, for example, the ability to perceive details or even the restricted interests of a child, could then become assets in some play situations.

Playing with others requires multiple skills, especially social skills. Through social play, children with autism learn about social interaction. Therapeutic and educational play settings should be designed to provide long-term learning processes. Before they can correctly express emotions in daily life, children with ASD need to learn to understand emotions and recognise them and their meaning. For this reason, *emotional recognition* and theory of mind are frequently taught to these children before work can begin to improve play for the sake of play (Thommen et al., 2010). Many social-cognition training programmes exist; they can be computerised (Silver, 2000 and Baron-Cohen, 2004 cited in Nader-Grosbois, 2011; Glaser et al., 2012 cited in Wood et al., 2013) or not (Howlin et al., 2010; Wellman et al., 2002). Social scenarios are also interesting tools for learning social interactions (Gray, 1994). However, in play situations, the child will be confronted with many different emotions and varied ways to express them, requiring direct application in everyday life contexts. Role-playing then seems a more appropriate tool for matching learnt social interactions to real life (Baghdadli & Brisot-Dubois, 2011).

Another way to intervene is illustrated with a study of 60 children with ASD in school integration situations, which compared interventions focussed on children with ASD versus their classmates (Kasari et al., 2012). When the intervention targeted the group of classmates, children with ASD were more often considered as members of the social network of the class than when the intervention was centred only on them. They became playing partners and were less frequently isolated during class breaks. Moreover, not only were changes observed in the attitudes of peers, but the social skills of the children with ASD also improved.

10.2 Types and Form(s) of Play Favoured by Children with ASD

According to Doody and Merz (2013), research examining the types of play favoured by children with ASD is limited. The understanding of the play preferences of children with developmental disabilities might be very challenging, particularly when they do not use the language consistently or do not have the cognitive ability for self-awareness.

Nevertheless, different features emerge when describing play among children with ASD: they often play with objects in a repetitive, restrictive, rigid, and non-symbolic manner, centred on sensorial particularities and/or on physical understanding. These features can be seen as a 'serious game' and a form of intentional play, as these children have such a thirst for knowledge. So, if we change our view on their activities, their play is rather a difference than a disability. For many children with ASD, 'banging a doll' or 'pouring sand in different containers' are activities that require directed and skilled actions and could be considered a form of play, as well as an occupation for its own sake (Spitzer, 2003). With these examples, the distinction between repetitive and not-directed behaviour is very thin. Moreover, when sensorial stimuli, which are not spontaneously part of play, are added to support the children's motivation and attention in play (e.g., multiple sound effects during the activity, lighting effects, sensory materials), this may increase the repetitiveness of their behaviours to the point of sensorial fascination and self-stimulation actions. This form of automatic behaviour may not meet the criteria for play as an intentional occupation and may lead to isolation. However, for ASD children with restricted play interests, play might be the opportunity to experience a lot of fun, to play with peers, or to join a group of children with the same concerns, for example, 'manga' or 'trains'.

Children with ASD encounter difficulties in occupying their leisure time. For them, 'free' time is often a period of stress, as they do not know what to do in such a non-structured time. A new trend of research and intervention focussing on 'how to occupy myself' in leisure is developing to improve their occupation during leisure time (Chan et al., 2014; Seward et al., 2014). In fact, the primary skills needed to occupy leisure time can be impaired in children with ASD. Children must be able to make choices between different kinds of play and to initiate behaviours with selected objects. It is, therefore, important to offer them real tools to help them deal with leisure time. As spare time is not much fun for them, it is also necessary to offer them activities they like, such as the sensory play they spontaneously choose.

We can also note that other types of play are very successful in leisure time, for instance, those related to new technologies. One of their advantages is their attractiveness (Wainer & Ingersoll, 2011; Shane & Albert, 2008). In fact, touch screens or playful interfaces are all assets that stimulate children's motivation. Moreover, the programmed, predictable, and emotionally neutral environments of new technologies are particularly appreciated by children with ASD (Shane & Albert, 2008; Ramdoss et al., 2012). "Computer-proposed tasks are clearly defined and promote the focus of attention by reducing the distractions caused by irrelevant sensory stimuli" (Murray, 1999, in Grossard & Grynszpan, 2015:67). With such devices, children can play during their free time and also learn in a fun way, but with the risk that excessive use can lead to confinement and social isolation (Durkin, 2010; Ramdoss et al., 2012).

Robot-assisted therapy (RAT) (Diehl et al, 2012) is a large growing research area about using technology in diagnostic, play, and learning of children with ASD (Robins et al, 2012). Several types of robots have been researched. Vehicle-like robot 'Labo-1' supporting children play and using robots as social mediators in order to interact with other people (Werry et al., 2001). Humanoid-shaped robots showed the most promising results (Wainer et al., 2014). Snowman-shaped robot 'Keepon' encourages joint attention (Kozima et al., 2007). Robot 'Bandit' elicits positive social responses like speech, interactions with robot (Feil-Seifer & Matarić, 2006). Robot doll 'Robota' engages children in imitative interaction play (Robins et al., 2006). Humanoid robot KASPAR "encourages interaction between the children and copresent adults as a salient mediating object and help children to learn about tactile social behaviour" (Wainer et al., 2014).

In conclusion, the play of children with ASD is especially different from that of typical children; however, "careful observations have often come to the conclusion that many kinds of play are less affected in autistic children than was expected" (Trevarthen et al., 1998:109).

10.3 Play Environment and Participation of Children with ASD

The socio-cultural context is known to have a fundamental role in a person's ability to participate in an activity such as play (Pierce, 2001). Children with ASD may engage in play that is personally meaningful, but not socially conform and well-accepted, and most of the research on play amongst children with developmental disorders describes "deficient normative activities" or "failure to engage in expected activities" (Spitzer, 2003:72). They behave remarkably differently when part of a peer group. The participation in play amongst children with ASD reflects the core features of the condition. It is complicated by persistent socio-communication deficits in attention, imitation, and social responsiveness (Sigman & Ruskin, 1999). They inconsistently respond to peers when the latter initiate play with them (Attwood et al., 1988). They also have limited use of joint attention and other nonverbal skills, as well as marked spoken difficulties to ask for objects, request information, and share emotions, which make them unsustainable in social play (Schuler, 2003). Even when they show active interest in playing, they seem strange to typically developing children because they behave and talk in an idiosyncratic way (Boucher & Wolfberg, 2003; Jordan, 2003; Wing & Attwood, 1987; Wolfberg, 2009). This kind of social interaction is often considered undesirable, and response from peers is a negative reinforcement. In circumstances of mutual avoidance, children with ASD are at high risk of being excluded by peers or often exclude themselves from peer interactions. Thus, the aloofness associated with children with ASD results largely from peer group responses to them (Wolfberg et al., 2012).

Indoor and outdoor free-time activities with peers, which allow children to experience enjoyment, are known to offer the best opportunities for all children to engage with their environment and have the best chance of ensuring their participation (Heah et al., 2006). Playing is essential for friendship (Theodorou & Nind, 2012). However, children with a disorder, such as ASD, spend more time in controlled and learnt activities with adults rather than with peers, which raises important psychosocial barriers, such as making friends with whom to play (Miller et al., 2010). Children with high-functioning autism experience friendship differently than typically developing children or people with another disorder. They have fewer friends, and the friends they do play with are usually peers also with a disorder. They report a lower quality of friendship with less intimacy and closeness than their typical peers (Petrina et al., 2014). Finally, research on the inner experience of participation in play for children with ASD is emerging and needs further investigation.

10.4 Conclusion

Children with ASD present sensorimotor, cognitive, and socio-emotional skills impairments that can hinder play, particularly social play. An examination of their play preferences and interventions centred on their play competence are still rare (Wolfberg et al., 2012). When professionals have to deal with the challenging behaviours and the lack of language of children with ASD, "play is more likely to be viewed as a luxury only to be targeted when more basic deficiencies have been remedied" (Wolfberg et al., 2012:59). However, play in early intervention solicits positive emotions in children and develops their interest in social interaction. Introducing play and designing appropriate play opportunities for children with ASD need to be the primary concerns for educators, clinicians, and parents.

References

American Psychiatric Association (APA) (2013). *Diagnostic and Statistical Manual of Mental Disorders*. Arlington, VA: American Psychiatric Publishing.

Attwood, A., Frith, U., & Hermelin, B. (1988). The understanding and use of interpersonal gestures by autistic and Down's syndrome children. *Journal of Autism and Developmental Disorders*, 18, 241–57.

Baghdadli, A., & Brisod-Dubois, J. (2011). *Entraînement aux habiletés sociales appliqué à l'autisme: guide pour les intervenants*. Paris, F: Elsevier Masson.

Baron-Cohen, S. (2004). The cognitive neuroscience of autism. *Journal of Neurology, Neurosurgery, Psychiatry*, 75, 945-958.

Benson, J., Nicka, M., & Stern, P. (2006). How does a child with sensory processing problems play. *The Internet Journal of Allied Health Sciences and Practice*, 4(4). Retrieved from: http://ijahsp.nova.edu/articles/vol4num4/benson.pdf.

Ben-Sasson, A., Hen, L., Fluss, R., Cermak, S., Engel-Yeger, B., & Gal, E. (2009). A meta-analysis of sensory modulation symptoms in individuals with autism spectrum disorders. *Journal of Autism & Developmental Disorders*, 39(1), 1-11.

Cairney, J. (2015). *Developmental Coordination Disorder and its Consequences*. Toronto, CDN: University of Toronto Press.

Case-Smith, J., & Clifford O'Brien, J. (2014). *Occupational Therapy for Children and Adolescents (7th edition)*. St. Louis, MO: Mosby.

Case-Smith, J., & Kuhaneck, H. M. (2008). Play Preferences of Typically Developing Children and Children with Developmental Delays between Ages 3 and 7 Years. *OTJR: Occupation, Participation and Health*, 28(1), 19-29.

Chan, J. M., Lambdin, L., Graham, K., Fragale, C., & Davis, T. (2014). A Picture-Based Activity Schedule Intervention to Teach Adults with Mild Intellectual Disability to Use an iPad During a Leisure Activity. *Journal of Behavioral Education*, 23(2), 247-257.

Chiarello, L. A., Huntington, A., & Bundy, A. (2006). A comparison of motor behaviors, interaction, and playfulness during motherchild and fatherchild play with children with motor delay. *Physical & Occupational Therapy in Paediatrics*, 26(1/2), 129-151.

Deci, E.L., & Ryan, R.M. (1985). *Intrinsic Motivation and Self-determination in Human Behavior.* New York, NY: Plenum.

Diehl, J., Schmitt, L., Villano, M., Crowell, C. (2012). The clinical use of robots for individuals with autism spectrum disorders: A critical review. *Research in Autism Spectrum Disorders*, 6, 249-262.

Dewey, D., Cantell, M., & Crawford, S. G. (2007). Motor and gestural performance in children with autism spectrum disorders, developmental coordination disorder, and/or attention deficit hyperactivity disorder. *Journal of the International Neuropsychological Society*, 13, 246-256.

Doody, K. R., & Mertz, J. (2013). Preferred Play Activities of Children with Autism Spectrum Disorder in Naturalistic Settings. *North American Journal of Medicine and Science*, 6(3), 128-133.

Durkin, K. (2010). Videogames and young people with developmental disorders. *Review of General Psychology*, 14(2), 122-144.

Feil-Seifer, D., & Matarić, M. (2008). Toward socially assistive robotics for augmenting interventions for children with autism spectrum disorders. *Experimental Robotics*, 54, 201-210.

Fisher, A. G., Murray, E. A., & Bundy, A. C. (1991). *Sensory Integration: Theory and Practice*. Philadelphia, PA: F. A. Davis.

Gray, C. (1994). *Nouveau Livre de Scenarios Sociaux*. Québec, CDN: Jenison Public Schools.

Green, D., Charman, T., Pickles, A., Chandler, S., Loucas, T., Simonoff, E., & Baird, G. (2009). Impairment in movement skills of children with autistic spectrum disorders. *Developmental Medicine & Child Neurology*, 51(4), 311-316.

Grossard, C., & Grynszpan, O. (2015). Entraînement des compétences assistées par les technologies numériques dans l'autisme : une revue. *Enfance*, 1, 67-85.

Heah, T., Case, T., McGuire, B., & Law, M. (2007). Successful Participation: The Lived Experience among Children with Disabilities. *Canadian Journal of Occupational Therapy*, 74(1), 38-47.

Howlin, P., Baron-Cohen, S., & Hadwin, J. (2010). *Apprendre aux enfants atteints d'autisme à comprendre la pensée des autres.* Bruxelles, B: De Boeck.

Jarrold, C. (2003). A Review of Research into Pretend Play in Autism. *Autism*, 7(4), 379-390.

Jordan, R. (2003). Social play and autistic spectrum disorders: A perspective on theory, implications and educational approaches. *Autism*, 7(4), 347-360.

Kaplan, B. J., N. Wilson, B., Dewey, D., & Crawford, S. G. (1998). DCD may not be a discrete disorder. *Human Movement Science*, 17(4-5), 471-490.

Kasari, C., Rotheram-Fuller, E., Locke, J., & Gulsrud, A. (2012). Making the connection: randomized controlled trial of social skills at school for children with autism spectrum disorders. *Journal of Child Psychology and Psychiatry,* 53(4), 431-439.

Kennedy-Behr, A., Rodger, S., & Mickan, S. (2013). A comparison of the play skills of preschool children with and without developmental coordination disorder. *OTJR: Occupation, Participation and Health*, 33(4), 198-208.

Kern, J. K., Trivedi, M. H., Garver, C. R., Grannemann, B. D., Andrews, A. A., Savla, J. S., ... & Schroeder, J. L. (2006). The pattern of sensory processing abnormalities in. *Autism*, 10(5), 480-494.

King, G., Gibson, B. E., Mistry, B., Pinto, M., Goh, F., Teachman, G., & Thompson, L. (2013). An integrated methods study of the experiences of youth with severe disabilities in leisure activity settings: the importance of belonging, fun, and control and choice. *Disability and Rehabilitation*, 36(19), 1626-1635.

Koegel, R. L., & Kern Koegel, L. (2006). *Pivotal Response Treatments for Autism: Communication, Social, and Academic Development.* Baltimore, MD: Paul H. Brookes Publishing.

Kozima, H., Nakagawa, C., & Yasuda, Z. (2007). Children-robot interaction: A pilot study in autism therapy. *Progress in Brain Research*, 164, 385-400.

Lane, S. J., & Bundy, A. C. (2012). *Kids Can Be Kids: A Childhood Occupations Approach.* Philadelphia, PA: F. A. Davis.

Lane, A. E., Young, R. L., Baker, A. E., & Angley, M. T. (2010). Sensory processing subtypes in autism: Association with adaptive behavior. *Journal of Autism and Developmental Disorders*, 40(1), 112-122.

Lovaas, O. I. (1987). Behavioral treatment and normal educational and intellectual functioning in young autistic children. *Journal of Consulting and Clinical Psychology*, 55(1), 3.

Luckett, T., Bundy, A., & Roberts, J. (2007). Do behavioural approaches teach children with autism to play or are they pretending?. *Autism*, 11(4), 365-388.

Miller Kuhaneck, H. M., Spitzer, S. L., & Miller, E. (2010). *Activity Analysis, Creativity And Playfulness In Pediatric Occupational Therapy: Making Play Just Right.* Mississauga, CDN: Jones & Bartlett Publishers.

Nadel, J. (2002). Imitation and imitation recognition: Functional use in preverbal infants and nonverbal children with autism. In A. N. Meltzoff, & W. Prinz (Eds) *The Imitative Mind: Development, evolution, and Brain Bases*, (pp. 42-62), Cambridge, UK: University Press.

Nader-Grosbois, N. (2011). *La Théorie de l'esprit.* Bruxelles, B: De Boeck.

Perrin, J. (2011). *Le jeu chez les enfants avec autisme.* Presented at the "Journée départementale: Autisme et Jeu". Tarbes, France.

Petrina, N., Carter, M., & Stephenson, J. (2014). The nature of friendship in children with autism spectrum disorders: A systematic review. *Research in Autism Spectrum Disorders,* 8(2), 111-126.

Pierce, D. (2001). Untangling occupation and activity. *American Journal of Occupational Therapy,* 55, 138-146.

Poulsen, A. A., & Ziviani, J. M. (2004). Can I play too? Physical activity engagement of children with developmental coordination disorders. *Canadian Journal of Occupational Therapy. Revue canadienne d'ergothérapie*, 71(2), 100.

Ramdoss, S., Machalicek, W., Rispoli, M., Mulloy, A., Lang, R., & O'Reilly, M. (2012). Computer-based interventions to improve social and emotional skills in individuals with autism spectrum disorders: a systematic review. *Developmental Neurorehabilitation,* 15(2), 119-35.

Robins, B., Dautenhahn, K., Ferrari, E., Kronreif, G., Prazak-Aram, B., Marti, P., ... & Laudanna, E. (2012). Scenarios of robot-assisted play for children with cognitive and physical disabilities. *Interaction Studies*, 13(2), 189-234.

Rogers, S. J., Hepburn, S., & Wehner, E. (2003). Parent Reports of Sensory Symptoms in Toddlers with Autism and Those with Other Developmental Disorders. *Journal of Autism and Developmental Disorders*, 33(6), 631-642.

Rogers, S. J., & Dawson, G. (2010). *Early Start Denver Model for young children with autism: promoting language, learning and engagement.* New York, NY: The Guilford Press.

Schaaf, R.C., & Mailloux, Z. (2015). *Clinician's guide for implementing Ayres Sensory Integration.* Bethesda, MD: AOTA Press.

Schaaf, R. C., Toth-Cohen, S., Johnson, S. L., Outten, G., & Benevides, T. W. (2011). The everyday routines of families of children with autism: Examining the impact of sensory processing difficulties on the family. *Autism*, 1-17.

Schopler, E. (1997). Implementation of TEACCH philosophy. *Handbook of autism and pervasive developmental disorders*, 2, 767-795.

Schuler, A. L. (2003). Beyond echoplaylia: Promoting language in children with autism. *Autism: International Journal of Research and Practice, 7*, 455–69.

Seward, J., Schuster, J. W., Ault, M. J., Collins, B. C., & Hall, M. (2014). Comparing Simultaneous Prompting and Constant Time Delay to Teach Leisure Skills to Students with Moderate Intellectual Disability. *Education and Training in Autism and Developmental Disabilities*, 49(3), 381-395.

Shane, H. C., & Albert, P. D. (2008). Electronic screen media for persons with autism spectrum disorders: Results of a survey. *Journal of Autism and Developmental Disorders*, 38(8), 1499-1508.

Sigman, M., & Ruskin, E. (1999). Continuity and change in the social competence of children with autism, Down syndrome, and developmental delays. *Monographs of the Society for Research in Child Development, 64*, 1-114.

Smyth, M. M., & Anderson, H. I. (2000). Coping with clumsiness in the school playground: Social and physical play in children with coordination impairments. *British Journal of Developmental Psychology*, 18(3), 389-413.

Spitzer, S. L. (2003). With and Without Words: Exploring Occupation in Relation to Young Children with Autism. *Journal of Occupational Science*, 10(2), 67-79.

Stanković, M., Lakic, A., & Ilic, N. (2012). Autism and autistic spectrum disorders in the context of new DSM-V classification, and clinical and epidemiological data. *Srp Arh Celok Lek*, 140(3-4), 236-243.

Tanta, K. J., & Knox, S. H. (2015). Play. In J. Case-Smith & J. Clifford O'Brien (Eds), *Occupational Therapy for Children and Adolescents (7th edition)* (pp. 483-495). St. Louis, MO: Mosby.

Ten Eycke, K. D., & Müller, U. (2015). Brief report: new evidence for a social-specific imagination deficit in children with autism spectrum disorder. *Journal of Autism and Developmental Disorders*, 45(1), 213-220.

Theodorou, F., & Nind, M. (2010). Inclusion in play: a case study of a child with autism in an inclusive nursery. *Journal of Research in Special Educational Needs*, 10(2), 99-106.

Thommen, E., Cartier-Nelles, A., Guidoux, A., & Wiesendanger, S. (2014). Les particularités cognitives dans le trouble du spectre de l'autisme: la théorie de l'esprit et les fonctions exécutives. *Swiss Archives of Neurology and Psychiatry*, 165(8), 290-297.

Thommen, E., Suarez, M., Guidetti, M., Guidoux, A., Rogé, B., & Reilly, J. S. (2010). Comprendre les émotions chez les enfants atteints d'autisme: regards croisés selon les tâches. *Enfance*, 3, 319-337.

Trevarthen, C., Aitken, K., Papoudi, D., & Robarts, J. (1998). *Children with Autism: Diagnosis and Intervention to Meet their Needs.* London, UK: Jessica Kingsley.

Wainer, A. L., & Ingersoll, B. R. (2011). The use of innovative computer technology for teaching social communication to individuals with autism spectrum disorders. *Research in Autism Spectrum Disorders*, 5(1), 96-107.

Wainer, J., Robins, B., Amirabdollahian, F., & Dautenhahn, K. (2014). Using the Humanoid Robot KASPAR to Autonomously Play Triadic Games and Facilitate Collaborative Play Among Children With Autism. *IEEE Transactions On Autonomous Mental Development*, 6(3).

Watling, R. L., Deitz, J., & White, O. (2001). Comparison of Sensory Profile Scores of Young Children With and Without Autism Spectrum Disorders. *American Journal of Occupational Therapy*, 55, 416-423.

Wellman, H. M., Caswell, R., Gomez, J. C., Swetthenham, J., Toye, E., & Lagattuta, K. (2002). Thought-bubbles help children with autism acquire an alternative to a theory of mind. *Autism*, 6(4), 343-363.

Werry, I., Dautenhahn, K., & Harwin, W. (2001). Evaluating the response of children with autism to a robot. In R. Simpson (Ed.), *RESNA Rehabilitation Engineering and Assistive Technology Society of North America Annual Conference* (pp. 14–19). Arlington, VA: Resna Press.

Wing, L., & Attwood, A. (1987). Syndromes of autism and atypical development. In: D. Cohen & A. Donnellan (Eds.), *Handbook of Autism and Pervasive Disorders*. New York, NY: John Wiley & Sons.

Wolfberg, P. J. (2009). *Play and Imagination in Children with Autism*. New York, NY: Teachers College Press.

Wolfberg, P., Bottema-Beutel, K., & DeWitt, M. (2012). Including Children with Autism in Social and Imaginary Play with Typical Peers. *American Journal of Play*, 5(1), 55-80.

Wood, H., Glaser, B., & Eliez, S. (2013). L'autisme: les nouveaux programmes thérapeutiques. *Swiss Archives of Neurology and Psychiatry*, 164(1), 13-19.

Francesca Caprino and Vittoria Stucci

11 Play in Children with Multiple Disabilities

11.1 Introduction

Play, a universal behaviour, documented in every culture, may have atypical characteristics in the child with multiple disabilities. The lack of access to sensorial inputs and the additional motor, cognitive, and communicative impairments observable in these children can cause a delay in all areas of development and may also lead to play behaviours that are not as rich as those of their peers.

Children with multiple impairments have enormous problems not only in receiving the multitude of stimulations coming from the environment, but also in properly decoding them. As a result, they experience a kind of 'chaotic misinformation' that may produce a sense of danger (Frohlich, 2007), and that massively interferes with the development of play skills.

Yet, in these cases, play has an even more important role with respect to a child with typical development (Brodin, 1999): through play, children can not only demonstrate their skills, but also acquire new ones in many areas of development.

Of particular importance is the relationship between the development of play skills and the development of communicative skills (Brodin, 1991; Pizzo & Bruce, 2010), an aspect that highlights the importance of play as a factor that gives the child with multiple disabilities the opportunity of relating with his or her environment.

It is for this reason that caring for a child with multiple disabilities must include activities that affect play; activities that aim not only at bringing out and strengthening the child's skills, but that are also capable of influencing the contexts in which the child interacts.

11.2 Play and Multiple Disabilities: the Literature

Most of the research on play in children with multiple disabilities focuses on the use of play as a tool for evaluating children's skills and as a strategy suitable for achieving educational or therapeutic objectives. For what concerns the use of play for assessment and diagnostic purposes, the quality of play is reported by the literature as a parameter capable of providing information about the degree of overall development of the child with multiple disabilities (Finn et al., 1988; Mar, 1996) or about specific aspects, such as the development of object permanence (Bruce, 2012) and language (Pizzo & Bruce, 2010).

While no tools for evaluating the play skills of this population have been specially validated or developed, some assessment tools designed for children with multiple disabilities do have items that refer to ludic behaviours and are used to observe the various components of the child's development. This is the case involving the Callier-Azusa scale (Stillman, 1978), a tool to evaluate the development of the deaf-blind child and with multiple disabilities that includes, in the subscales that refer to the degree of perceptive, motor and social development, numerous behavioural items that describe play activities involving practice play (e.g., grabbing and shaking objects, throwing, rolling, bouncing, and catching a ball), construction play (e.g., stacking blocks, handling Plasticine, cutting, colouring), symbolic play (e.g., presence of pretend play), and play with rules. The INSITE developmental checklist for multihandicapped sensory-impaired infants and young children (Morgan et al., 1999), used with children up to six years of age, includes numerous items that refer to observation of play activities.

The literature relative to the use of play as a tool for achieving educational or rehabilitative objectives, in particular in early interventions aimed at infants and young children, refers to the research in which the ludic activity is utilised to improve perception skills and to increase residual sensorial functions, movement (Lieberman & Tolla, 2000), communication (Michael, 1990), socialisation with peers (Hanline & Correa-Torres, 2012), and cognitive development (Fleer, 2014).

A major line of research investigates the role of play in rehabilitative–behavioural activities aimed at reducing maladaptive behaviours (self-injury, aggressiveness, self-stimulation). According to the so-called communication paradigm, these behaviours are nonverbal forms of communication aimed at obtaining gratifying environmental responses (Emerson, 2001) and can be replaced with more appropriate and functionally equivalent conduct, such as simple activities involving manipulation of objects or toys (Lancioni & O' Reilly, 2010). As a result, this allows the child to reach the same objectives sought with inappropriate behaviour while expanding his or her behavioural repertoire at the same time.

In recent years, above all, in the occupational therapy environments (Pharam & Fazio, 2008) and also thanks to the research and intervention initiatives developed by specialised centres for children with multiple disabilities and their families, approaches that encourage the development of the ludic factor, considered as an objective in itself and capable of positively affecting all aspects of the child's development and quality of life, have been rather successful.

11.3 Impairments in Functions Linked with Play and Ludic Activities

Children with multiple disabilities have congenital or acquired impairments in one or both sensorial channels, that can be associated to a severe development and intellectual delay, motor deficits, severe behavioural disturbances, and other dysfunctions linked to additional organic pathologies that are neurological or of other origins.

Deaf-blindness,[1] meaning the combination, with different degrees, of sight and hearing impairments not associated with other disabilities, can be considered a condition in and of itself. In these cases, generalised problems arise due to sensorial distortions that make interaction with the environment more difficult. Such difficulties, however, are not as severe compared with those encountered by children who have additional motor or cognitive impairments. In the presence of multiple disabilities, it always becomes necessary to develop educational and rehabilitative interventions that are specific from a methodological and instrument perspective. In some cases, some developmental milestones considered essential for the general development and for the emergence of play abilities were not achieved: these may include joint attention (Nunez, 2014), turn taking, or understanding of cause–effect relationships (Finn et al., 1988).

Children with multiple disabilities may exhibit unusual responses when presented with objects or activities, take a lot of time to process stimuli, or on the contrary, exhibit excessive, intense, and at times, even violent activities with forms of self- or other-directed aggressiveness.

Spontaneous ludic behaviours often involve maladaptive responses: these children have very low motor responsiveness levels in the presence of gratifying stimuli, stereotypical behaviours apparently independent from adaptive purposes, and the tendency to use the object for self-stimulation (Coppa et al. 2005; Nisi & Ceccarani, 1993).

Social skills may be severely compromised and require specific action that guides the child to overcome his or her isolation. In more serious cases, it becomes necessary to start from the development of awareness of the presence of others to arrive gradually, in situations with a high level of structuring, at establishing positive interactions.

In general, for cases involving multiple disabilities, there are not only low levels of initiative and exploration, but also less involvement in symbolic and cooperative play.

11.4 The Role of the Environment for Participating in Play Activities

Due to the previously described factors, participation by children with multiple disabilities in play activities typical for their age may be very limited. This reduced degree of participation is not attributable, however, only to personal impairments,

---

1 According to the Declaration of the European Parliament on the Rights of Deaf-Blind People (2004), "deaf-blindness is a distinct disability that is a combination of both sight and hearing impairments, which results in difficulties having access to information, communication and mobility". http://www.europarl.europa.eu/sides/getDoc.do?pubRef=-//EP//TEXT+TA+P5-TA-2004-0277+0+DOC+XML+V0//EN&language=SL

but also to the characteristics of the living environments. Parents of children with multiple disabilities often feel they are incapable of playing with their children (Brodin, 1999). Early interactions in the mother-child dyads are particularly critical. In their research from 2007, Coppa and Orena observed that the mothers of children with multiple disabilities tend to fill all the empty spaces of the ludic interaction with hyper-stimulatory behaviours. The same authors also point out how the exchanges are characterised by communicative expressions of the mother, especially verbal ones. In addition, the mothers find it difficult to get in synch with their children and tend not to leave space to process the stimulus, demonstrating a tendency to normalise the interaction.

The characteristics of the play spaces may also represent a barrier. Factors such as lack of access to play areas and playgrounds and the presence of potentially disturbing factors (such as noise, insufficient lighting) can also make a difference in terms of opportunities to participate in play activities. Additional participation problems may be due to the unavailability of play materials that are suitable, adapted, or specifically designed for play and leisure time of infants and young children with multiple disabilities.

Play participation opportunities are also strictly correlated to the degree of inclusion of the child with multiple disabilities in school and in his or her community, to the possibility of playing with peers with or without disabilities, and to the presence of support from services that utilise professionals with specific training for this complex type of disability. It is these services that play a critical role in providing information and advice to parents and in guiding them, through a working alliance, to get in synch with their children in various pleasurable play activities.

11.5 Facilitating Play in Children with Multiple Disabilities

Children with multiple disabilities, under proper conditions, can utilise the richness of the ludic experience, and with it, reach significant development objectives, provided that there are facilitating contexts: the most important factors are the relationship with the adult and the type of toys and structure of the overall physical context (Brodin, 1991). Another crucial factor is selecting the play materials (Brodin, 1999). Indeed, such a selection must be based on specific observations of the child and correspond to his or her specific perceptive, cognitive, motor, and communicative characteristics, as well as his or her preferences. There are numerous types of materials starting with simple tactile exploration games (such as containers filled with different materials: water, sand, balls, etc.). The child, using enjoyable and comfortable procedures, must be able to safely perceive, understand, and manipulate the materials and with minimal help (Canalini et al., 2005). If necessary, specific assistive technologies can also be used, such as switches that allow children with motor or sensory impairments to activate a toy through alternative methods.

In selecting toys and playware, it is important to consider the degree of accessibility and the presence of enhanced sensory characteristics, such as acoustic, visual, tactile, or gustatory feedback (food can also be an excellent play material); it is also important to encourage the child to choose and explore the proposed material (Coppa et al., 2005).

With children who exhibit behavioural stereotypes or who use specific objects for which there would seem to be a strong stereotyped attraction, it could be useful to propose similar materials within the context of activities that may develop into functional learning. If, for example, the child spends a lot of time on self-stimulating activities, that is, passing the hands in front of the eyes, play activities should contain strong visual elements, such as lights that turn on and off, software with cause–effect activities with dazzling visual feedback, and so on.

Observation, a key element of the intervention involving play skills, must be carried out possibly within the daily living contexts and with the help of professionals who can correctly interpret the child's responses when presented with the proposed materials. In particular, satisfaction with the proposed play activities can be evaluated through systematic measurement of positive reactions, that is, of 'happiness indices' (Dillon & Carr, 2007).

The 'indices of happiness' are used to evaluate the level of pleasure and wellness in persons without language skills by measuring easy-to-observe behaviours (e.g., laughing, smiling, clapping hands) correlated with inner emotional states. Some research has shown how these manifestations can be actively increased by modifying the environment and that their frequency increases, in particular during play activities. It is important to consider, when observing such indicators, that each child can express his or her wellness in a subjective manner and that the responses may occur much later than those exhibited by children with typical development.

The physical and perceptive characteristics of spaces and their organisation also play an important role: in addition to being accessible, spaces must also be capable of stimulating the child and providing a suitable range of possible activities (Brodin & Lindstrand, 2006).

To increase the child's independent exploration, play environments should be designed and organised so that their function is immediately recognisable: it is possible, for example, to create paths and dividing lines of the play areas using materials with contrasting colours and different types of roughness, or by using elements with olfactory clues, selecting and arranging the furniture to reduce sensory and cognitive obstacles to a minimum (Canalini et al., 2005).

For infants, small ludic environments (a play corner) can be created in which materials provide auditory, visual, tactile, and olfactory stimuli and where the child, according to a non-directive approach, can move freely and enjoy the proposed experience.

When setting up the activities in the play corner, it is important to carefully select the stimuli (chosen based on the observation of the child's preferences) and to create a rigorous path for learning the prerequisites necessary for interacting with the various elements that 'enrich' the environment.

Constant monitoring, always based on observation, will make it possible to measure the attention and pleasure maintenance level of the play corner stimuli.

Because adults play a fundamental role, they can motivate, provide models, as well as help and support ludic activities.

Of particular importance, especially in younger children, is the physical vicinity of the mother (Brodin, 1991), a figure that can promote early experiences of fundamental importance for the development of play skills. The first thing that the child plays with is his or her body, but to do this, it is necessary to be familiar with it and to be capable of locating each part.

The child with multiple disabilities does not easily become aware of what is around him or her therefore, a guide, even physical, is needed to encourage him or her to explore and experiment. The caregiver can facilitate the child to experience his or her body, helping him or her to touch own parts, stimulating and proposing play actions (ball pit play, rocking games) or relaxing activities (e.g., playing in water).

Finally, to overcome the problems that many parents have when playing with their children, it is important to provide support that facilitates their ability to observe and to enter in contact with their children, helping them to propose stimulating activities and to interact in the most appropriate manner, without replacing them.

When developing the rehabilitation project, the various professionals must maintain a constant channel of communication with the child's reference figures. Caring for the child with multiple disabilities must include care for the entire family and the use of an 'ecological' approach that will affect all contexts of the child's everyday life.

11.6 Conclusion

Even children with multiple disabilities can play, making independent choices, enjoying what they do and not expecting any reward, except the pleasure of playing itself. However, in many cases, free and self-determined play must be considered not as a starting point, but as an objective to achieve, creating even highly structured activities that accompany the child as he or she learns increasingly complex play skills, and adopting measures that will have a positive effect on the characteristics of the environment.

Given the heterogeneity of the motor, linguistic, intellectual, and sensorial characteristics of children with multiple disabilities, the intervention must be highly individualised and be based on specific observations of individual behaviour in family contexts and at different times (Gleason, 2008). Similarly, environmental changes must be personalised while also taking into account a child's progress and development.

References

Brodin, J., & Lindstrand, P. (2006). *Inclusion of children in Outdoor Education. Learning in Motion. Report I*. Stockholm, S: Stockholm Institute of Education.

Brodin, J. (2005). Diversity of aspects on play in children with profound multiple disabilities. *Early Child Development and Care*, 175(7), 635-646.

Brodin, J. (1999). Play in Children with Severe Multiple Disabilities: Play with toys - a review. *International Journal of Disability, Development and Education*, 46 (1), 25-34.

Brodin, J. (1991). *Att tolka barns signaler. Gravt utvecklingsstörda flerhandikappade barns lek och kommunikation* [Interpreting children's signals. Play and communication in children with profound mental retardation and multiple disabilities]. Stockholm, S: Stockholm University, Department of Education.

Bruce, S., & Vargas, C. (2012). Assessment and Instruction of Object Permanence in Children with Blindness and Multiple Disabilities. *Journal of Visual Impairment & Blindness*, 106(11), 717-727.

Canalini, R., Ceccarani, P., Storani, E., & Von Prondzinski, S. (2005). *Spazi incontro alla disabilità. Progettare gli ambienti di vita nelle pluriminorazioni sensoriali* [Spaces towards disability. Designing life environments for the sensorial multiple disabilities]. Trento, I: Erickson.

Chantry, J., & Dunford, C. (2010). How do computer assistive technologies enhance participation in childhood occupations for children with multiple and complex disabilities? A review of the current literature. *The British Journal of Occupational Therapy*, 73(8), 351-365.

Coppa, M., Orena, E., & Orlandoni M. L. (2005). Giochi e giocattoli per bambini pluriminorati: idee e percorsi educativi per la crescita della relazione intersoggettiva. In: *Proceedings of the V conference "La Qualità dell'Integrazione Scolastica"*. Trento, I: Erickson.

Dillon, C. M., & Carr, J. E. (2007). Assessing indices of happiness and unhappiness in individuals with developmental disabilities: A review. *Behavioral Interventions*, 22(3), 229-244.

Emerson, E. (2001). *Challenging behaviour: Analysis and intervention in people with severe learning disabilities*. Cambridge, UK: Cambridge University Press.

Finn, D., Fewell, R., & Vadasy, P. (1988). The play of young children who have dual sensory impairments. In: M. Bullis, & G. Fielding (Eds.), *Communication development in young children with deafblindness: Literature review* (pp. 149-163). Monmouth, OR: Oregon State System of Higher Education, Teaching Research Division.

Fleer, A. G. (2014). *An evaluation of the Cognitive Objects Play Intervention for children with profound multiple disabilities at a children's Home and three daycare centers in South Africa*. Utrecht, NL: Utrecht University.

Fröhlich, A. (2007). *La Stimolazione Basale per bambini, adolescenti, e adulti con pluridisabilità* [Basal stimulation for children, adolescents and adults with multiple disabilities]. Pisa, I: Edizioni del Cerro.

Gleason, D. (2008). *Early Interactions with Children Who Are Deaf-Blind*. National Consortium on Deaf-Blindness. Retrieved from: http://files.eric.ed.gov/fulltext/ED531843.pdf.

Hanline, M. F., & Correa Torres, S. M. (2012). Experiences of Preschoolers with Severe Disabilities in an Inclusive Early Education Setting: A Qualitative Study. *Education and Training in Autism and Developmental Disabilities*, 47(1), 109-121.

Lancioni, G. E., O'Reilly, M. F., Singh, N. N., Sigafoos, J., Didden, R., Oliva, D., & Campodonico, F. (2010). Two children with multiple disabilities increase adaptive object manipulation and reduce inappropriate behavior via a technology-assisted program. *Journal of Visual Impairment & Blindness*, 104(11), 714-719.

Lieberman, L. J., & Pecorella M. (2006). Activity at home for children and youth who are deafblind. *Deaf-Blind Perspectives*, 14(1), 3-7.

Lieberman, L. J., & MacVicar, J. M. (2003). Play and recreation habits of youth who are deaf-blind. *Journal of Visual Impairment and Blindness*, 97(12), 755-768.

Lieberman, L. J., & Brockport, S. (1996). Adapting Games, Sports, and Recreation for Children and Adults who are Deaf-Blind. *Deafblind perspectives*, 3(3), 5-8.

Mar, H. (1996). *Psychological Evaluation of Children Who Are Deaf-Blind: An Overview with Recommendations for Practice*. DB-LINK, Hellen-Keller National Centre for Deaf-Blind Youth and Adults, New England Region.

Michael, M. G., & Paul, P. V. (1990). Early intervention for infants with deaf-blindness. *Exceptional children*, 57(3), 200-210.

Morgan, E. C., Watkins S., Terry, B. G., Snow, P. S., Boyle, P., Watts, J., . Morrison, A, Jensen, D. L. (1989). *Insite developmental checklist*. North Logan, UT: HOPE.

Nisi, A., & Ceccarani, P. (1993). La valutazione psico-educativa nel portatore di handicap grave e di minorazioni multiple. Guida ai progressi del bambino [Psycho-educational evaluation of the person with severe and multiple disabilities]. *Hd-Handicap e disabilità di apprendimento*, 52, 1-48.

Nunez, M. (2014). *Joint attention in deafblind children: A multi-sensory path towards a shared understanding of the world*. Sense, Glasgow, UK: Glasgow Caledonian University.

Parham, L. D., & Fazio L. S. (2008). *Play in occupational therapy for children*. St. Louis, MO: Mosby.

Pizzo, L., & Bruce, S. M. (2010). Language and play in students with multiple disabilities and visual impairments or deaf-blindness. *Journal of Visual Impairment & Blindness*, 104(5), 287-297.

Reid, D. H., DiCarlo, C. F., Schepis, M. M., Hawkins, J., & Stricklin, S. B. (2003). Observational assessment of toy preferences among young children with disabilities in inclusive settings: Efficiency analysis and comparison with staff opinion. *Behavior Modification*, 27(2), 233-250.

Stillman, R. (1978). *The Callier-Azusa Scale*. Dallas, TE: Callier Center for Communication Disorders.

Sylvie Ray-Kaeser and Helen Lynch

12 Occupational Therapy Perspective on Play for the Sake of Play

Despite play being identified as being a core aspect of occupational therapy (OT) from as early as 1922, the focus on play receded and did not come to the fore again until research and writings from therapists, such as Mary Reilly (1974), and further work that came from the emergence of the new science of occupation in the 1980s and 1990s (Hocking, 2009). The resurgence of occupation coupled with global influences, such as the evolving ICF (WHO, 2001) and ICF-CY (WHO, 2007), has resulted in a shift away from the traditional biomedical model to an occupational model; practice is orienting more towards participation than body function and structure (Figure 12.1). Participation in play is related to an interaction between the children's motivation and abilities, the characteristics of the environment, and available activities matching their preferences (Figure 12.1).

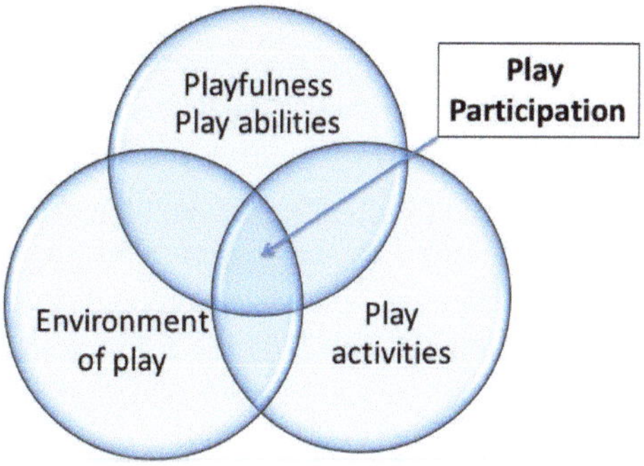

Figure 12.1. Focus on participation in play

An OT perspective on play is closely intertwined to the study of play from an occupational science perspective. Hence, this overview of the contribution of OT to play includes the study of play as an occupation (occupational science) as well as the translation of this knowledge into practice (OT). In occupational science and OT, *play* is named as a core element in the classification systems of occupations across the lifespan. It is viewed as the most common occupation of children, and *playing* one of the many daily routines, such as dressing, eating, and showering. Being a *player* is the primary occupational role of a child. Play is any fun activity that produces a sense of joy in the participant; it is viewed as a way of being, a state of mind, called *playfulness* (Lane & Bundy, 2012). Play is significant because it gives children a sense of mastery (Reilly, 1974), it transcends life's' distresses (Sutton-Smith, 2008), and it is central to how children learn, especially in the early years (Bateson, 2011).

Multiple disciplinary perspectives provide a strong basis for the theory of play as an occupation (Parham 2008). These include cognitive, psychodynamic, anthropological, motor, psychological, social, and competence fields of study. Researchers have built on these disciplinary perspectives to form an occupational therapy perspective specifically that reflects a *biopsychosocial view of play*. Research on play in the occupational science literature includes considering play in terms of occupational behaviour (Reilly, 1974) and play as occupational development (Humphry, 2002; Wiseman et al., 2005), integrating research on different play types and purposes, along with the influences of the physical and social environment on play (Knox, 1996; Pierce et al., 2009; Schneider, 2009).

From a *body function and structure* perspective, play is regarded as an important aspect of child development, consisting a variety of movements and manipulation of the environment: through play, the child develops sensory integration, physical, cognitive, and language skills (Tanta & Knox, 2015).

In relation to *activity and participation*, play includes a sociocultural perspective, where it is acknowledged that play is viewed and valued differently according to cultural values, customs, and norms (Bazyk et al., 2003; Parham, 2008). Studies of children with disabilities have found that these children experience social exclusion in play activities due to difficulties in joining similar physical play activities as their peers (Law et al., 2013; Poulsen et al., 2007).

Regarding the *environment*, the physical environment is known to have a significant influence on the occupational development of the child (Lynch, 2012; Pierce, 1996). Researchers have found that the physical environment shapes play (Lynch, 2009; Prellwitz & Skar, 2007) and that playfulness is influenced by the environment (Rigby & Huggins, 1997). Concerning systems and policy contexts, play is considered as an occupational justice issue and a fundamental occupational right (Wilcock & Townsend, 2000). Conditions such as play deprivation, inability to engage in play, exclusion from play activities, and inaccessibility to playgrounds or other play spaces can be alleviated through social or political actions (Moore & Lynch, 2015).

Overall, play is a *quality of life* issue, improving the health and wellbeing of communities, groups, and individuals (Parham, 1996). Play as healing exercises "cognitive and affective flexibility to aid resilience", which is "central to human adaptability" (Dell Clark, 2015:375). Play serves adaptation and has an adaptive function. It is believed to facilitate inclusion, social participation, and flexibility in thinking, learning, and problem-solving (Stagnitti & Unsworth, 2000).

While occupational science research values the extrinsic functional contribution of play to child development, it also values the intrinsic contribution for the child: "play is a vehicle for meaning" (Parham, 1996:78). Through interviews or observation with children and their families, the subjective meaning of play occupation has been studied (Prellwitz, 2007; Spitzer, 2003a; Tamm & Skar, 2000). While the subjective meaning for the child may not always be apparent, using an occupational science approach to understand play helps us to see that it is the individual's experience of the activity that determines whether it is enjoyable (Pierce, 2001; Spitzer, 2003b).

To summarise, an occupational perspective of play is that it "only occurs when there is a 'just right' fit between the child and the environment" (Cooper, 2009:33), that it can be both productive as well as pleasurable and that it can be embedded in obligatory tasks and requires effort (Humphry, 2002). While play may be defined as pleasurable, it can still be productive, and therefore, there is no dilemma in arguing that play is also "serious business" (Bruner, 1976:20).

12.1 Definition of Play from the Discipline of OT

Play is defined in OT as any spontaneous or organised child-directed activity that is an interaction between the child and the environment, which "provides enjoyment, entertainment, amusement or diversion" (Parham & Fazio, 2008:448). It is characterised by core elements: intrinsic motivation, where the child is free to engage; controlled by the player; freedom from external rules or direction; with attention on the play process rather than on the product of play (Rigby & Rodger, 2006; Skard & Bundy, 2008). Although it is viewed as providing amusement and diversion, it should not be confused with being frivolous; it is the means through which the child learns and develops, the source of wellbeing, and is consequently an aspect of childhood that requires serious consideration. The American Association of OT (AOTA) acknowledges the importance of play in its "Societal Position on Play (Primeau, 2008:707):

> *OT practitioners support, enhance, and defend children's right to play as individuals and as members of their families, peer groups, and communities by promoting recognition of play's crucial role in children's development, health, and wellbeing; establishing and restoring children's skills needed to engage in play; adapting play materials, objects, and environments to facilitate optimal play experiences; and advocating for safe, inclusive play environments that are accessible to all.*

12.2 Play in OT (how OT Contributes to the Topic)

Play has a central place in OT as primary means and goals for intervention with children (Parham & Fazio, 2008). This means that play in OT may not be play at all: it is often addressing functional skills for play or utilising a playful approach to target other skills (play as a means to an end). OT is also concerned with making sure that the child's basic needs are met, so that they are able to play (e.g., environmental adaptations). Consequently, Bundy (2011) considers that there are five facets of play that have particular relevance to OT practice with children and families:

1. Skills for play
2. Approach to play (play attitude)
3. Play activities
4. Environmental supportiveness for play
5. Source of motivation for play

The occupational therapists (OTs) base their intervention on their knowledge of these five facets, with specific attention to play activities and characteristics (form, function, meaning, and context), of the art of play and science of human occupation (Hinojosa & Segal, 2012). They closely analyse how intra-individual characteristics and environments support or interfere with play to generate multiple therapeutic strategies at three levels of service.

1. *Universal*
- Assisting in the promotion of play for all children through the development of policies.
- Educating the community on the importance of play.
- Advocating a universal design for the public play areas and equipment.

2. *Targeted*
- Providing play environments usable for children at risk of developing health challenges.
- Assessing, selecting, and adapting play materials, equipment, toys, and games.
- Providing assistive technology for play for the 'at risk' group of children.

3. *Intensive*
- Encouraging child-parent playful interactions and educating families to balance their time with playful activities.
- Enabling engagement in play and play inclusion of a child with disability.
- Expending a child's cognitive, physical, social, emotional, and play skills through individualised intervention.

The OTs provide *assessment* of a child's play and playfulness, although play assessments have a limited role to date in OT practice (Miller Kuhaneck et al., 2013). As play typically occurs in the child's environment, play assessment requires tools that facilitate an accurate and authentic assessment in context; therefore, observation of unstructured play in context is most common (Bundy, 2011) with observational tools such as the Test of Playfulness (ToP) (Skard & Bundy, 2008) as well as the environmental supportiveness of the player's motivation for play (TOES) (Bronson & Bundy, 2001). Other forms of assessment include parent interviews about the play experiences of their child (Play History, Takata, 1974; Initial interview with parents, EIP, Ferland, 2003) or interview with the child (Pediatric Interest Profiles, PIP, Henry, 2000; Pediatric Activity Card Sort, PACS, Mandich et al., 2004). They also assess the play behaviour of a child (Revised Knox Preschool Play scale, RKPPS, Knox, 2008; Child Initiated Pretend Play, CHIPPA, Stagnitti, 2007; Evaluation of ludic behaviour in children, ECL, Ferland, 2003). To date, no assessment has been developed in OT for assessing motivation for play, and this has been noted as being an aspect requiring further research (Bundy, 2011).

OT *intervention* for play can be in the form of play as means versus ends (McLaughlin Gray, 1998) and play as both means and ends. In each case, where OT is working directly with the child, the therapist can utilise varied approaches that can be considered as a continuum from a teaching approach (non-play), to directed play, to guided play, and then free play (Table 12.1).

Table 12.1. Continuum from therapist initiated to child-initiated play (adapted from Henrick, 2015 and Wood, 2007)

Relationships OT-child in play	**Therapist-initiated and directed**	**Therapist-initiated or child-responsive**	**Child-initiated or therapist-scaffolded and guided**	**Child-initiated, child-led, and child-directed**
Kind of activity	Activities are taught and practised	Activities are playful or play-based	Activities are playful, play-based, self-chosen, and voluntary	Activities are intrinsically motivated, self-chosen, voluntary
Kind of play	Work or non-play	Directed play i.e., playful work	Guided play, i.e., work-like play	Free play

← ← ← ←......moving from extrinsic motivation to intrinsic motivation.......... → → →

Play as means to an end. The OTs use spontaneous and/or organised play as an attractive tool or medium to act upon the primary consequences of the disability and/or prevent psychosocial difficulties. They use playful activities to improve specific skills, which are expected to develop abilities in a range of daily activities. In this form of intervention, the child is directed to using play objects and play activities, in order to enable the development of specific motor, sensory, cognitive, emotional, and social skills. The child may not have a choice in the activity and may have less control in the play than if it was freely chosen and self-directed. Hence, the play form in this mode of intervention is more typically oriented towards directed, adult-led activity, to support learning. Play is primarily used in this instance as a motivator for engaging the child in therapy (Bundy, 2011; Miller Kuhaneck et al., 2013). Play as a means to an end refers, therefore, to playful activities rather than play.

It is known that interventions using playful activities yield better results than repeated exercises, for example, to increase the range of movement of children with burn injuries (Melchert-McKearnan et al., 2000). There is evidence that playful motor intervention with children at risk of developmental delay provides positive outcomes (Fromberg & Bergen, 2015). The OTs use objects' and toys' motivational properties to increase the appeal of therapeutic activities, address common performance skills, and support engagement in occupation. They create therapeutic situations in which children can experiment new skills with fewer risks and use play to encourage children's participation.

Play as a therapeutic medium is also used outside clinical contexts, working, for example, in the family home in response to traumatic events or child's inner conflicts (Johnson et al., 2015). More recently, play interventions have been developed to address obesity and increasing physical activity in childhood through playground design (Bundy et al., 2008; Bundy et al., 2011; Engelen et al., 2013).

Play as ends/goal. When the OTs use play as the goal, this takes on many forms: the OT may consider addressing play skills of the child or addressing social and physical environmental enablers for play.

One OT intervention where activities, such as play, can be the goal is *the Cognitive Orientation to Daily Occupational Performance* (CO-OP) programme (Polatajko & Mandich, 2004). In this cognitive intervention, the therapist supports the child to identify and explore new strategies for learning a desired skill, such as riding a bike through problem-solving and practising in weekly therapy sessions. When play is the goal, the intervention uses playful activities rather than self-directed play; the child does not engage in a form of play that is flexible, where he or she can move from one activity to another at will. Instead, the child focuses on the chosen play activity and through directed engagement and guided discovery (i.e., guided by the OT), practises new strategies for successful achievement of the activity. An example of specific OT intervention where play is the goal is the *Learn to Play* programme from Australia, where the therapist begins by using a directed play approach until the child becomes more competent in play skills and moves to guided play (Stagnitti, 2004). The focus of this programme is to enable adults to direct the child in pretend play, beginning with the child's developmental level and modelling the play activity. The child is encouraged to develop six core skills: sequence of play actions, object substitution, play scripts, doll/teddy play, social interaction, and role play (Stagnitti, 2009). In a more recent work, further developments in play-based approaches have expanded to include interventions for children with ADHD, in home contexts and incorporating parents and friends in the therapy process (Wilkes-Gillan et al., 2014). Each example of intervention approaches demonstrates the current move towards contextual, participatory methods in provision of play-based OT, with a strong focus on changing the environment as a way to enable play.

The OTs include goals related to environmental supportiveness for play and skills for play aimed at improving play participation of children with special needs, enhancing parent-child interactions and play access. They can help families that struggle to manage their complex daily occupations with a child with disabilities. They identify the strategies the parents use at home to manage their child and support them to find and use the most appropriate ones for integrating play into the life of the whole family. They use their knowledge to adapt play and play materials. In such a family-centred approach, intervention is not always specifically aimed at reaching specific goals for the child only, but also for the parents and child to play without assistance from the therapist (Lane & Bundy, 2012).

The OTs also enable all children to play and promote playfulness and spontaneous, active community play experiences for children for the value of free play for its own sake (Lane & Bundy, 2012). This is in adherence with the overarching outcome of OT to promote engagement in occupation to support participation. They use their knowledge to notice play inequities. They address the children's engagement in play within the context of their lives, the home, school, and community (Parham & Fazio, 2008). They support the parents to engage fully with their children through play and avoid play deprivation knowing that the actual hurried lifetime, the changes in family structures, and increased attention to organised extra-scholar activities reduce the time for free play in families (Singer et al., 2009). They support teachers and educators to create play opportunities in the school and day-care environment, in school playgrounds, as many schools restrict the play by removing play equipment and break time (Bundy et al., 2008; Ramstetter et al., 2010).

Combining play as means and play as ends. In other OT interventions, play is utilised as both a means to an end and also as the goal. One example of this is an OT intervention called *Ayres Sensory Integrative approach* (ASI), which provides opportunities for children with sensory-processing disorders to engage in active, child-led, and child-driven playful and fun activities with achievable challenges in a secure (safe) environment (Schaaf & Miller, 2005). This is an example where intervention is required to be play-based and the child is facilitated to engage in physical activity play primarily, through child-initiated, therapist-responsive activities. In this form of intervention, the child is not fully engaging in free play, but is more accurately taking part in guided play, where the therapist sets up the environment, so that the child will choose certain play activities (Weisberg et al., 2013). It is a form of guided play that meets their developmental needs and is based on the intrinsic motivation of the child (Table 12.2).

12.3 Conclusion

OTs are in a unique position to promote play for children in general and for children with disabilities, creating opportunities for an inclusive environment of play and providing education on the need for play to promote a healthy and playful life. To date, few studies have examined the effectiveness of using different approaches to play in intervention: to compare the effect of directed-play versus guided play versus free-play in enabling play occupation. Yet, in educational studies, play-based learning has been shown to be more effective than direct instruction, especially for pre-schoolers (Hirsh-Pasek et al., 2009). More research is needed to explore the different forms of play-based intervention, and specifically, the place of guided play or free-play as an effective means of enabling participation in play occupations for children with disabilities. If free play is the serious work of the child, then we must ensure that play occupation is more central in our work, as part of our role in enabling play as ends, and not just considering play as a means to an end.

References

Bateson, P. (2011). Theories of play. In A. Pellegrini (Ed.), *The Oxford Handbook of the Development of Play* (pp. 41-47). Oxford, UK: Oxford University Press.

Bazyk, S., Stalnaker, D., Llerena, M., Ekelman, B., & Bazyk, J. (2003). Play in Mayan children. *American Joural of Occupational Therapy,* 57(3), 273-283.

Bronson, M., & Bundy, A. (2001). A correlational study of the test of playfulness and the test of environmental supportiveness. *Occupational Therapy Journal of Research*, 21, 241-259.

Bruner, J. (1976). Introduction. In J. Bruner, A. Jolly & K. Sylva (Eds.). *Play: its Role in Development and evolution* (pp. 13-27). Harmondsworth, UK: Penguin Books.

Bundy, A. (2011). Children: analysing the occupation of play. In L. Mackenzie & G. O'Toole (Eds.), *Occupation Analysis in Practice (1st ed.)* (pp. 133-146). Oxford, UK: Blackwell Publishing ltd.

Bundy, A. C., Luckett, T., Naughton, G. A., Tranter, P. J., Wyver, S. R., Ragen, J., ... & Spies, G. (2008). Playful interaction: Occupational therapy for all children on the school playground. *American Journal of Occupational Therapy*, 62(5), 522527.

Bundy, A. C., Naughton, G., Tranter, P., Wyver, S., Baur, L., Schiller, W., ... & Brentnall, J. (2011). The Sydney playground project: popping the bubblewrap - unleashing the power of play: a cluster randomised controlled trial of a primary school playground-based intervention aiming to increase children's physical activity and social skills. *BMC Public Health,* 11, 1-9.

Cooper, R. (2009). Play as transaction: The impact of child maltreatment. In K. Stagnitti & R. Cooper (Eds.). *Play as Therapy: Assessment and Therapeutic Interventions.* (pp. 176-186). London, UK: Jessican Kingsley Publishers.

Engelen, L., Bundy, A., Naughton, G., Simpson, J., Bauman, A., Ragen, J., ... & Van der Ploeg, H. (2013). Increasing physical activity in young primary school children—it's child's play: A cluster randomised controlled trial. *Preventative Medicine*, 319-325.

Ferland, F. (2003). *Le modèle ludique (3ème ed.).* Montréal, CDN: PUM.

Fromberg, D. P., & Bergen, D. (2015). *Play from Birth to Twelve: Contexts, Perspectives, and Meanings.* New York, NY: Routledge.

Henrick, T. (2015). *Play and the Human Condition.* Chicago, IL: University of Illinois Press.

Henry, A. D. (2000). *Paediatric Interest Profiles: Surveys of Play for Children and Adolescents, Kid Play Profile, Preteen Play Profile, Adolescent Leisure Interest Profile.* Psychological Corporation, a Harcourt Assessment Company.

Hinojosa, J. & Segal, R. (2012). Building intervention from theory. In S. J. Lane & A. C. Bundy (Eds.), *Kids Can Be Kids: A Childhood Occupations Approach* (pp. 161-179). Philadelphia, PA: F. A. Davis.

Hirsch-Pasek, K., Golinkoff, R., Berk, L. & Singer, D. (2009). *A Mandate for Playful Learning in Preschool; Presenting the evidence.* New York, NY: Oxford University Press.

Hocking, C. (2009). The challenge of occupation: describing the things people do. *Journal of Occupational Science,* 16(3), 140-150.

Humphry, R. (2002). Young children's occupations: explicating dynamics of developmental processes. *American Journal of Occupational Therapy,* 56, 171-179.

Dell Clark, C. (2015). Play interventions and therapy. In J. E. Johnson, S. G. Eberle, T. S. Henricks, & D. Kuschner (Eds), *The Handbook of the Study of Play* (pp. 365-380). London, UK: Rowman & Littlefield Publishers.

Knox, S. (1996). Play and playfulness in preschool children. In R. Zemke & F. Clark (Eds), *Occupational Science: the evolving Discipline* (pp. 81-88). Philadelphia, PA: F. A. Davis.

Knox, S. (2008). Development and current use of the Revised Knox Preschool Play Scale. In L. D. Parham & L. Fazio (Eds), *Play in Occupational Therapy for Children (2nd ed.)* (pp. 55-70). St Louis, MO: Mosby Elsevier.

Lane, S. J., & Bundy, A. C. (2012). *Kids Can Be Kids: A Childhood Occupations Approach.* Philadelphia, PA: F. A. Davis.

Law, M., Anaby, D. Teplicky, R., Khetani, M.A., Coster, W., & Bedell, G. (2013). Participation in the home environment among children and youth with and without disabilities. *British Journal of Occupational Therapy,* 76(2), 58-66.

Lynch, H. (2009). Patterns of activity of Irish children aged five to eight years: City living in Ireland today. *Journal of Occupational Science*, 16(1):44-49.

Lynch, H. (2012). *Infant Places, Spaces and Objects: Exploring the Physical in Learning Environments for Infants Under Two.* (Doctoral dissertation). Dublin Institute of Technology, Dublin.

Mandich, A., Polatajko, H., Miller, L. & Baum, C. M. (2004). *The Paediatric Activity Card Sort (PACS).* Ottawa, CDN: Canadian Occupational Therapy Association.

McLaughlin Gray, J. (1998). Putting occupation into practice: Occupation as ends, occupation as means. *American Journal of Occupational Therapy,* 52, 354-364.

Melchert-McKearnan, K., Deitz, J., Engel, J. M., & White, O. (2000). Children with burn injuries: Purposeful activity versus rote exercise. *American Journal of Occupational Therapy,* 54, 381-390.

Miller Kuhaneck, H., Tanta, K., Coombs, A. & Pannone, H. (2013). A survey of paediatric occupational therapists use of play. *Journal of Occupational Therapy, Schools & Early Intervention*, 6, 213-227.

Montessori, M. (1967). *The Absorbent Mind.* New York, NY: Holt, Rinehart & Winston.

Moore, A., & Lynch, H. (2015). Accessibility and usability of playground environments for children under 12: A scoping review. *Scandinavian Journal of Occupational Therapy*, 22(5), 331-344.

Parham, L. D. (1996). Perspectives on play. In R. Zemke & F. Clark (Eds.), *Occupational Science: the evolving Discipline* (pp. 71-80). Philadelphia, PA: F. A. Davis.

Parham, L. D. (2008). Play and occupational therapy. In L. D. Parham & L. Fazio (Eds.), *Play in Occupational Therapy for Children (2nd ed.)* (pp. 219-249). St Louis, MO: Mosby Elsevier.

Parham, L. D., & Fazio, L. S. (2008). *Play in Occupational Therapy for Children.* St-Louis, MO: Mosby Elsevier.

Pierce, D. (1996). *Infant space, infant time: development of infant interactions with the physical environment, from 1 to 18 months.* Doctor of Philosophy Doctoral thesis, University of Southern California, Los Angeles.

Pierce, D. (2001). Untangling occupation from activity. *American Journal of Occupational Therapy,* 55(2), 138-146.

Pierce, D., Munier, V., & Teeters-Myers, C. (2009). Informing early intervention through an occupational science description of infant-toddler interactions with home space. *American Journal of Occupational Therapy,* 63(3), 273-287.

Polatajko, H., & Mandich, A. (2004). *Enabling Occupation in Children: The Cognitive Orientation to Daily Occupational Performance (CO-OP) approach.* Ottawa, ON: CAOT Publications.

Poulsen, A. A., Ziviani, J. M., & Cuskelly, M. (2007). Perceived freedom in leisure and physical co-ordination ability: impact on out-of-school activity participation and life satisfaction. *Child: Care, Health and Development*, 33(4), 432440.

Prellwitz, M. (2007). *Playground Accessibility and Usability for Children with Disabilities.* PhD thesis: Lulea University of Technology, Sweden.

Prellwitz, M., & Skar, L. (2007). Usability of playgrounds for children with different abilities. *Occupational Therapy International,* 14(3), 144-155.

Primeau, L. (2008). AOTA's societal statement on play. *American Journal of Occupational Therapy,* 62(6), 707-708.

Ramstetter, C. L., Murray, R., & Gardner, A. S. (2010). The crucial role of recess in schools. *Journal of School Health,* 80(11), 517-526.

Reilly, M. (1974). *Play as exploratory Learning*. Beverly Hills, CA: Sage Publications.
Rigby, P., & Huggins, L. (1997). Enabling young children to play by creating supportive play environments. In L. D. Parham & L. Fazio (Eds.), *Play in Occupational Therapy (1st ed.)*, (pp. 155-176). St. Louis, MO: Mosby.
Rigby, P., & Rodger, S. (2006). Developing as a player. In S. Rodger & J. Ziviani (Eds.), *Occupational Therapy with Children: Understanding Children's Occupations and enabling Participation* (pp. 177-199). London, UK: Blackwell.
Schaaf, R. C., & Miller, L. J. (2005). Occupational therapy using a sensory integrative approach for children with developmental disabilities. *Mental Retardation and Developmental Disabilities Research Reviews*, 11(2), 143–148.
Schneider, E. (2009). Longitudinal observations of infant object play behaviour in the home context. *OTJR: Occupation, Participation & Health*, 29(2), 79-87.
Singer, D., Singer, J., D'Agostino, H., & DeLong, R. (2009). Children's pastimes and play in sixteen nations : Is free play declining? *American Journal of Play*, 1, 283-312.
Skard, G., & Bundy, A. (2008). Test of Playfulness. In L. D. Parham & L. Fazio (Eds.), *Play in Occupational Therapy for Children* (pp. 71-93). St. Louis, MO: Mosby Elsevier.
Spitzer, S. (2003a). With and without words: exploring occupation in relation to young children with autism. *Journal of Occupational Science*, 10(2), 67-79.
Spitzer, S. (2003b). Using participant observation to study the meaning of occupations of young children with autism and other developmental disabilities. *American Journal of Occupational Therapy*, 57(1), 66-76.
Stagnitti, K. (2004). Occupational performance in pretend play: Implications for practice. In M, Mollineux (Ed.). *Occupation for Occupational Therapists* (pp. 103-121). Oxford, UK: Blackwell Science.
Stagnitti, K. (2007). *The Child-Initiated Pretend Play Assessment: Manual and Kit.* Melbourne: Co-ordinates Therapy Services.
Stagnitti, K. (2009). Play intervention-The Learn to Play Program. In K. Stagnitti & R. Cooper (Eds.), *Play as Therapy: Assessment and Therapeutic Interventions.* (pp. 176-186). London, UK: Jessican Kingsley Publishers.
Stagnitti, K., & Unsworth, C. (2000). The importance of pretend play in child development: An occupational therapy perspective. *The British Journal of Occupational Therapy*, 63(3), 121127.
Sutton-Smith, B. (2008). Play Theory: a Personal Journey and new Thoughts. *American Journal of Play*, 80-123.
Takata, N. (1974). Play as a prescription. In M. Reilly (Ed.), *Play as exploratory Learning* (pp. 209-246). Beverly Hills, CA: Sage Publications.
Tamm, M., & Skar, L. (2000). How I play: roles and relations in the play situations of children with restricted mobility. *Scandinavian Journal of Occupational Therapy*, 7(4), 174-182.
Tanta, K. & Knox, S. (2015). Play. In J. Case-Smith & J. Clifford O'Brien (Eds.), *Occupational Therapy for Children and Adolescents (7th ed.).* (pp. 483-493). St. Louis, MO: Elsevier Mosby.
Weisberg, D. S., Hirsh-Pasek, K., & Golinkoff, R. M. (2013). Guided Play: Where Curricular Goals Meet a Playful Pedagogy. *Mind, Brain, and Education*, 7(2), 104-112.
Wilcock, A., & Townsend, E. (2000). Occupational terminology interactive dialogue. *Journal of Occupational Science*, 7(2), 84–86.
Wilkes-Gillan, S., Bundy, A., Cordier, R. & Lincoln, M. (2014). Child outcomes of a pilot parent-delivered intervention for improving the social play skills of children with ADHD and their playmates. *Developmental Neurorehabilitation*, early online, 1-8.
Wiseman, J. O., Davis, J. A., & Polatajko, H. J. (2005). Occupational development: towards an understanding of children's doing. *Journal of Occupational Science*, 12(1), 26-35.
Wood, E. (2007). New directions in play: consensus or collision? *Education*, 3(13), 309-320.

World Health Organisation–WHO (2001). *International Classification of Functioning Disability and Health*. Geneva, CH: WHO.
World Health Organisation (2007). *International Classification of Functioning Disability and Health, Children and Youth Version*. Geneva, CH: WHO.

Michele Mainardi

13 Contribution of Special Education to the Promotion of Play for the Sake of Play

13.1 Introduction

Thanks to play, a child, for what concerns his or her personality as well as learning and self-assertion tools, can develop his or her identity and discover and exert his or her own power of free and intentional action on the environment and on persons, on relationships between subjects who play and on things. Play situations are certainly one of the opportunities where the chid enjoys the pleasure of competence. Discovery, emergence, and differentiation of interests and abilities are some of the basic factors in the play activity and of its intrinsic underlying motivation (Santer et al., 2007). Success and pleasure provide incentives for and orient motivation. Conversely, 'resistance to assimilation', 'difficult access', and failure can be first factors of exclusion and dependence, and then, of anger, frustration or resignation, and renouncement (learned helplessness).

13.2 Development of the Child, Developmental Disability, Special Education

Every child has innate and early skills that allow him or her to have certain forms of interaction with the surrounding physical and social world (Vygotskij, 1978). The 'state of development' of a person depends on countless factors. It is the end result of his or her behaviours, internal events (such as beliefs, expectations, self-perception, goals, intentions, physical structures, sensory and neural systems), and the effect of external factors, including social influences, roles in society, and the physical environment (Bandura, 1992).

The results and manifestations of development are the product of an indefinable quantity of processes. All individuals develop continually in their own way and at their own pace (Shaffer et al., 2002); consequently, "everyone has a unique developmental trajectory and outcome" (Skelton & Rosenbaum, 2010: 1).

This concept of development, and of the numerous factors influencing such growth, has led special education to focus increasingly on how and under what conditions an ability can be developed, and on how a disability can be managed in the interest of a person's global development, acting independently on the facilitators, and obstacles to development and to the opportunity of doing something, so that each person can develop and act to the best of his or her abilities, regardless of his or her distance from or reference to standards (World Health Organisation, 2002).

Special education operates where the concepts of development disability and child development intersect, but there are still many unanswered questions about such an intersection (Rosenbaum, 2008; Rosenbaum, 2009; Skelton & Rosenbaum, 2010).

13.3 Development and Play in Special Education

Play must be considered a process that embraces a wide range of abilities, motivations, behaviours, social situations, environments, contexts, and opportunities (Moyles, 2005).

A child who plays draws great benefit from this activity (Caffari-Viallon, 1988; Hewes, 2006; Selleck, 2001; Sheridan, 1977); however, not all have the same play opportunities at either a quantitative or qualitative level. This depends on the various obstacles or facilitators encountered in the context where the person develops. These obstacles and facilitators, interacting with a person's abilities and developmental disabilities, can disturb or favour the play activities just like they disturb or favour his or her daily habits, placing the child in a situation offering complete opportunity or, on the contrary, a handicap (Fougeyrollas, 1995; Rosenbaum, 2008).

In special education, more than anywhere else, play is often subordinated to other education or developmental priorities, or proposed according to forms and modalities that with regard to the ludic activity traditionally recognise strengths that can be used to enhance the attractiveness and effectiveness of rehabilitative or compensatory learning activities (Saracho & Spodek, 1998, 2003).

Less frequently than others, a child with disabilities finds himself or herself in situations that put him or her in the condition to play spontaneously, with pleasure and in complete freedom (with regard to time and method). Rubin et al. (1983) summarise the distinctive criteria of the play activity as follows. Play is: (1) intrinsically motivated (not governed by appetitive drives, compliance with social demands, or by inducements external to the behaviour itself); (2) controlled by the players (spontaneous, free from external sanctions, its goals are self-imposed); (3) concerned with a process rather than product (play asks "What can I do with this object or person?", and this question differentiates play from exploration that asks, "What is this object/person and what I do with it/him/her?"); (4) non-literal (play activities can be labelled as pretence); (5) free of externally imposed rules (this distinguishes play from games with rules); and (6) characterised by active engagement of the players (this distinguishes play from daydreaming, lounging, and aimless loafing). Therefore, it is not enough that an activity has the characteristic features of play to be considered as ludic.

What makes play unique and richer is the simultaneous presence of each of the factors indicated in this definition; their impact on the development of a child with a development disability, on his or her experience in taking action in different situations, and on the freedom to undertake such action; the emergence of subjectivity and differentiation of the intrinsic motivation in taking action; testing the possibility of playing. In education, attention aimed at the uniqueness of the child with some impairments in his or her relationships with the world and with learning qualifies special education. The attention focused on the characteristics of the child with disabilities, on the educational environment, and on the play opportunities (adequacy and accessibility) by special education qualify the consideration that the latter has for play by children with disabilities.

13.4 Spontaneous Play in Special Education

An absolute priority in special education is to concentrate on free and spontaneous play as a learning and development factor and on accessibility of experience opportunities as a condition of the experience (Aufauvre, 1980; Loos & Hoinkis, 2001; Mainardi, 2010; Santer et al., 2007). Play is important for all children. Special education must ensure that children with disabilities have the same opportunities to play as everyone else: "Self-determination is an educational outcome" (Wehmeyer, 1996). The studies that focus on this issue (Nankervis & Stancliffe, 2006; Wehmeyer & Garner, 2003; Wehmeyer et al., 2003) show that self-determination is directly correlated to the opportunities to make choices supported by the environment.

Educational contexts within which children with special education needs develop must take into account that "Self-initiated free play experiences are vital for the normal growth and development of all children" (Missiuna & Pollock, 1991: 882). The adequacy of the environment, the accessibility of the situations and of the play opportunities, and the frequency of the experience affect the possibility of experiencing play and oneself in play.

The specific educational context with special consideration for (1) the individual child, (2) accessibility of the living and development environment, and (3) the predisposition of opportunities for choice and free action determine the play opportunities and must be the focus of attention of education professionals and education consultants of families of children with disabilities. The child who due to endogenous, educational, or environmental reasons cannot carry out active roles in play situations, involving responsibility of choice and management of activities, is a child with a disadvantage (Bronfenbrenner & Ceci, 1994).

According to Bronfenbrenner (1992), personal attributes have the power to influence psychological and social development ("developmentally instigative personal characteristics") just like the "hierarchical environmental system of influence" in which the person is inserted, as well as time.

Sontag (1996), based on the considerations by Shonkoff et al. (1992), states that the influence on the development by exogenous factors at the base of a disability (organic causes of genetic or environmental origin) is important, but it has been proven that the environmental characteristics contribute significantly to a child's skills. The psychomotor competences of the child significantly affect the behavioural manifestations, and in particular, spontaneous play, adaptive behaviours, and mother-child interactions.

The type and degree of disabilities, as such, are not predictive indicators of instigator characteristics of a person's specific development. The characteristics of a child generally associated with development include health problems (heart and neurological disorders), personality traits, and their behavioural manifestations; the convictions of family members as far as how and what influences the enrichment of a child's development; instead, neither gender nor general family characteristics (family structure, economic situation, profession, health, ethnic group, etc.) would seem to have an influence as specific instigator factors.

Other studies (Zetlin et al., 1987) report how some adults (parents or education professional) exert too much control on the child (hyperprotection, priority on interventions based on education, and development purposes aimed at acquiring specific instrumental skills), while others assume different attitudes, more open to the independent and self-initiated experience. Other research studies confirm the reduction in expectations towards independent activity of the child with disabilities by the adult in relation with the decreased initiative and reaction times (Eheart, 1982; Gunn et al., 1982; Jones, 1977; Serpa & Meneres, 2003).

Physical, social, personal, and environmental barriers that limit the play experiences of children with disabilities must be delineated and considered in a facilitatory approach to the promotion of free play at home and at school (Missiuna & Pollock, 1991). Children with disabilities may find themselves in a situation with an accumulation of difficulties due to (1) greater dependence on their caregivers compared to other children; (2) spending more time than their peers at home; (3) passive involvement in activities made necessary by possible requests to provide the person with assistance. In addition, parents who are called on to act as a therapist with the child have less time and are less inclined to prepare and accompany free play situations, especially if they are not considered as particularly significant activities within the PEP (Personalised Education Plan).

Special education must consider that children with developmental disabilities may have a disadvantage in the exploration, interaction, and use of experience and play opportunities. There may be an impairment in the activity that allows the child to discriminate play, and therefore, take full advantage of the experiences through the senses and movement (Goldschmied & Jackson, 1994; Hutt et al., 1989; Karrer et al., 1979; Mainardi 1988; Ryan & Jones, 1975).

With respect to spontaneous and free play opportunities, special education must prevent the additional accumulation of difficulties (secondary impairments) in children with disabilities (Mainardi, 2013). To do this, special education must consider the 'handicap',[1] that the child must or can cope with (Mainardi, 2010). Attention with regard to the accessibility of opportunities and the adequacy of toys, situations, and play materials must be focused on the child's deficits and subsequent functional limitations. The presence of disabilities has a more or less direct effect on the quality and quantity of play opportunities and on their possible impact on a child's development.

The objective difficulties that the child encounters in the development process represent the source, that is, the initial stimulus of the manifestation of compensatory processes (Barisnikov & Petitpierre, 1994), but at the same time, the objective disabilities of the child motivate the compensatory activities also with his or her entourage.

The presence of disabilities in a child must not, in any case whatsoever, lower the level of expectations with respect to the importance of play, the inherent pleasure of play, and the opportunities of playing. The caregivers (from parents to professionals) must force themselves to allow the child to play and must intervene with caution in moments perceived as impasses in the play activity not to compensate, but to respect and promote the child's intentionality and action.

It is of little importance if a child has a disability or not, the child must play. To do this, it is important that the child has time, that there are playmates, and that he or she is given space and accessibility to the environment; that the surrounding social entourage enjoys playing, watching someone play, teaching to play, and considers the importance of play for the development of the person who is playing.

13.5 "Let me (them) Really Play": a Priority in Special Education

The risk that play is suffocated by other concerns or by 'compensatory' activities that, with regard to play are merely instigative without having other important and specific characteristics, exists to the extent in which the educational professional, the family, and peers act as if it were enough to let children play. A child's play must be motivated, safeguarded, and developed in all cases, but even more so, for the case involving children with a handicap.

It is of vital importance that whoever is close to the child should not only focus on compensating for a deficiency or a disability (Harrist & Bradley, 2003). It is crucial to think of the child. The impairment must be bypassed, so that the child can take full advantage of his or her condition, just like any other child:

1 In special education, the purpose behind the notion of handicap is to be able to distinguish, in operative terms, the influencing factors that make it possible to provide specific references to the mediation and support activity to facilitate accessibility of experience opportunities, from the general condition of the person with a disability (Mainardi, 2010).

1. Free and spontaneous play is the right of every child, as is the possibility of being able to fully exploit adequate and accessible play opportunities (at a physical, cognitive, affective, and social level).
2. The child with some type of impairment must be able to have the chance to play with satisfaction and success: he or she must be able to distinguish the opportunities and the specific characteristics of the free play situations and to experience and to exercise his or her abilities to intervene on the development and management phases of the play sequence as a fact and event in his or her life.
3. Play situations must be adaptated and made accessible (Mainardi, 2010) and must allow the child with some type of impairment to be included within his or her natural social context and his or her group of peers.

Special education must have the following educational priority: "Of prime importance for play, however, are the relationships that the adult develops, which give children the confidence to act autonomously, make choices, follow their interests and interact with peers. In other words, creating a context in which children feel psychologically safe and socially included" (Santer et al., 2007:59).

References

Aufauvre, M. H. (1980). *Apprendre* à jouer, apprendre à vivre. Le jeu, le jouet pour l'enfant handicapé: option pédagogique et thérapeutique. Paris, F: Delachaux & Niestlé.

Bandura, A. (1992). Social cognitive theory. In R. Vasta (Ed.), *Six Theories of Child Development: Revised Formulations and Current Issues* (pp. 1-60). Philadelphia, PA: Jessica Kingsley Publishers.

Barisnikov, K., & Petitpierre, G. (1994). *Vygotsky. Défectologie et déficience mentale* [Vygotskji. Defectology and mental deficit]. Neuchâtel, CH & Paris, F: Delachaux et Niestlé.

Bronfenbrenner, U. (1992). Ecological Systems Theory. In R. Vasta (Ed.), *Six Theories of Child Development: Revised Formulations and Current Issues* (pp. 187-250). Philadelphia, PA: Jessica Kingsley Publishers.

Bronfenbrenner, U., & Ceci, S. J. (1994). Nature-nurture reconceptualized in developmental perspective: A bioecological model. *Psychological Review*, 101, 568-586

Caffari-Viallon, R. (1988). *Pour que les enfants jouent*. Lausanne, CH: éditions EESP.

Eheart, B. (1982). Mother-child interaction with nonretarded and mentally retarded preschoolers. *American Journal of Mental Deficiency*, 87, 20-25.

Fougeyrollas, P. (1995). Documenting environmental factors for preventing the handicap creation process: Quebec contributions relating to ICIDH and social participation of people with functional differences. *Disability and Rehabilitation*, 17(3-4), 145-153.

Goldschmied, E., & Jackson, S. (1994). *People under Three*. London, UK: Routledge.

Gunn, P., Berry, P., & Andrew, R. (1982). Looking behavior of Down syndrome infants. *American Journal of Mental Deficiency*, 87, 344-347.

Hutt, S., Tyler, S., Hutt, C., & Christopherson, H. (1989). *Play, Exploration and Learning: A Natural History of the Pre-school*. London, UK: Routledge.

Jones, O. (1977). Mother-child communication with pre-linguistic Down's syndrome and normal infants. In: H. Schaffer (Ed.), *Studies in Mother, Infant Interaction*. London, UK: Academic Press.

Karrer, R., Nelson, M., & Galbraith, G. C. (1979). Psychophysiological research with the mentally retarded. In: N. J. Ellis (Ed.), *Handbook of Mental Deficiency, Psychological Theory and Research* (pp. 231-288). Hillsdale, NJ: Erlbaum.
Loos, S., & Hoinkis, U. (2001). *Handicap? Anche noi giochiamo!* [Handicap? We play too!]. Torino, I: Edizioni Gruppo Abele.
Mainardi, M. (1988). Comportement exploratoire et apprentissage. In: L. Lambert (Ed.), *Enfants et adultes handicapés mentaux. Recherches et applications*. Fribourg, CH: DelVal.
Mainardi, M. (2013). L'apport de la "defectologie moderne" aux pédagogies: en deçà de la Zone Proximale de Developpement (ZPD). In: J. P. Bernié, & M. Brossard (Eds.), *Vygotskij et l'école*. Pessac, F: Presses Universitaires de Bordeaux.
Missiuna, C. & Pollock, N. (1991). Play Deprivation in Children With Physical Disabilities: The Role of the Occupational Therapist in Preventing Secondary Disability. *American Journal of Occupational Therapy*, 45, 882-888.
Moyles, J. (2005). *The Excellence of Play*. Maidenhead, UK: Open University Press.
Nankervis, K. & Stancliffe, R. (2006). Supporting empowerment and choice making. In: I. Dempseyand, & K. Nankervis (Eds.), *Community Disability Services: An evidence-Based Approach to Practice* (pp. 81-109). Sydney, AUS: UNSW Press.
Serpa, J., & Menéres, S. (2003). The development of children with down syndrome: the influence of maternal adaptation, mother-child interaction and early forms of support. *European Journal of Special Needs education*, 18(2), 209-225.
Rosenbaum, P. (2008). Effects of powered mobility on self-initiated behaviours of very young children with locomotor disability (1986). *Developmental Medicine & Child Neurology*, 50(9), 644-644.
Rubin, K. H., Fein, G., & Vandenberg, B. (1983). Play. In E. M. Hetherington (Ed.), *Handbook of Child Psychology: Vol 4. Socialization, Personality, and Social Development*. New York, NY: Wiley.
Ryan, M., & Jones, B. (1975). Stimulus persistence in retarded and non retarded children. *American Journal of Mental Deficiency*, 80, 298-305.
Saracho, O. N., & Spodek, B. (1998). *Multiple Perspectives on Play in Early Childhood Education*. New York, NY: State University of New York Press.
Saracho, O. N., & Spodek, B. (2003). *Contemporary Perspectives on Play in Early Childhood, Vol. III*. Greenwich, CT: Information Age Publishing.
Selleck, D (2001). Being under 3 years of age: Enhancing quality experiences. In G. Pugh (Ed.) *Contemporary Issues in the Early Years: Working Collaboratively for Children*. London, UK: Paul Chapman Publishing.
Sheridan, M. (1977). *Spontaneous Play in Early Childhood: from Birth to Six Years*. Windsor, UK: NFER.
Shonkoff, J., Hauser-Cram, P., & Upshur, C. (1992). Development of infants with disabilities and their families: Implications for theory and service delivery. *Monographs of the Society for Research in Child Development*, 57.
Skelton, H., & Rosenbaum, P. (2010). *Disability and Child Development: Integrating the Concept*. CanChild, Centre for Childhood Disability Research. Retrieved from: https://www.canchild.ca/en/resources/35-disability-and-child-development-integrating-the-concepts.
Sontag, J. C. (1996). Toward a Comprehensive Theoretical Framework for Disability. *The Journal of Special education*, 30, 319-344.
Vygotskij, L. S. (1978). *Mind and society*. Cambridge, MA: Harvard University Press.
Wehmeyer, M. (1996). Self-determination as an educational outcome: Why is it important to children, youth and adults with disabilities? In D. J. Sands, & M. L. Wehmeyer (Eds.), *Self-Determination across the Life Span: Independence and Choice for People with Disabilities* (pp. 15-34). Baltimore, MD: Paul H. Brookes Publishing.

Wehmeyer, M., & Garner, W. (2003). The impact of Personal Characteristic of People with Intellectual and Developmental Disabilities on Self-determination and Autonomous Functioning. *Journal of Applied Research in Intellectual Disabilities*, 16, 225-265.

Wehmeyer, M., Abery, B., & Stanclife, R. (2003). *Theory in Self-Determination: Foundation for educational Practice*. Springfield, IL: Charles C. Thomas.

World Health Organization (2002*). Towards a Common Language for Functioning, Disability and Health: ICF.* Geneva, CH: WHO.

Zetlin, A., Turner, J., & Winik, L. (1987). The role of attention in retardate discrimination learning. In N. R. Ellis (Ed.), *Handbook of Mental Deficiency* (pp. 159-223). New York, NY: Mc-Graw-Hill.

Vaska Stancheva-Popkostadinova and Tatjana Zorcec

14 Play in Early Intervention for Children with Disabilities

14.1 Introduction

Early intervention is described as a system designed to support family patterns of interaction that best promote child development (Guralnick, 2001), consisting in multidisciplinary services provided to children from birth to five years of age (Shonkoff & Meisels, 2000).

Blackman sustains that "the goal of early [childhood] intervention is to prevent or minimise the physical, cognitive, emotional, and resource limitations of young children with biological or environmental risk factors" (2003:2).

Numerous studies emphasise the benefits of early intervention in the process of achieving developmental targets and goals for children with disabilities. Play has a central role in early intervention for children with disabilities, and it is used both for assessment and intervention. Some researchers regard play as a developmental domain, some as a medium for the development of specific skills (Bergen, 1987), while the others consider play as a domain for assessment, intervention, and curriculum activities (Lifter et al., 2011) in the process of delivering intervention procedures aimed at improving the a child's developmental and learning abilities (Casby, 2003; Lifter, 2008; Linder, 1993; Nwokah et al., 2013; Pierce, 1997).

Adults often use playtime to help children learn and often demand that play is functional to scopes other than fun. Obviously, learning is really important, but adults must not forget that when children play, 'function' is not what they are looking for. Children are simply playing and having fun. We know that play is intrinsically motivated and children are strongly determined to do this activity. When adults attempt to structure and direct the children's play, sometimes their intervention can be stressful and children can respond rebelliously (Sutton-Smith, 1987). Needless to say, adults must support play, facilitate and promote positive play. This support is especially beneficial for children with developmental delays.

14.2 Play in Early Intervention

One of the first extended overviews concerning the use of play in early intervention was proposed by Doris Bergen, who made an interesting review of the existing literature on the "suggested uses of play for assessment, prevention, and intervention with special needs children" (Bergen, 1991:1). The vision and proposals she stressed are still actual: play-based model of assessment conducted by a trans-disciplinary team; advantages and recommendations for overcoming the disadvantages of uses of play in early intervention for children with disabilities.

The use of play as a context for assessment and intervention and as a vehicle for successful inclusion in early care and educational settings intensified in the 1990s (Buchanan & Johnson, 2009). In their analysis of the use of play in early intervention, Lifter et al. (2011) delineated two important benefits of play for children with disabilities: facilitation of the development of more advanced play skills and the provision of a natural playful context to make it easier important clinical activities, such as the assessment and the implementation of educational and rehabilitation activities with a wide variety of goals in different developmental areas.

Early intervention programmes for children with disabilities are generally based on three different approaches: behavioural, developmental, and a combination of both. While the first approach is mainly addressed to implement new abilities in the child through specific 'ad hoc' plans of intervention, the last two are more related to the use of play and will briefly discussed in what follows.

The *developmental approach* is generally play-based and carried out in the child's natural environment. While adults play an integral part when applying the methodologies related to this approach, they do not actively structure or lead the learning opportunity. Play-based approaches to learning support the concept of natural environments presented in the early intervention literature (Dunst, 2007; Dunst & Bruder, 2002; Hanft & Pilkington, 2000). Play activities are used to implement goals in a variety of developmental domains (Sandall et al., 2005) for child-focussed interventions (Wolery, 2005).

Several studies have provided evidence of systematic relationships between developments in play and developments in other domains (Lifter et al., 2011). The integration of activities addressed to teach new skills into the play routines can be effective in improving both play and other developmental domains (Dunst, 1981).

Combined programmes have been developed using principles from both the behavioural and developmental approaches. In what follows, some example are shortly presented.

The Early Start Denver model promotes learning through play in natural routines, in combination with structured teaching techniques associated with behavioural therapies; it aims at developing play skills and language abilities (Rogers & Dawson, 2010). TEACCH (Treatment and Education of Autistic and related Communication handicapped CHildren) is an intensive intervention programme to promote learning and development, in particular, in the areas of communication and social skills, independence, coping skills, and skills for daily life. Children are supported by creating a very structured learning environment (Peeremboom, 2003). JASPER (Joint Attention Symbolic Play Engagement Regulation) targets the foundations of social communication (joint attention, imitation, play), uses naturalistic strategies to increase the rate and complexity of social communication, and includes parents and teachers as implementers of the intervention to promote generalisation across settings and activities and to ensure maintenance over time (Kasari et al., 2012).

14.3 Play-based Assessment

Assessment of development of sensorimotor and social play, as well as the onset, quantity, and quality of symbolic play in children can give indications about the possible delays in other developmental domains, and may support and validate other assessment measures that denote developmental problems (Bergen, 1991).

Play-based assessment occurs either in a special setting that has been designed to elicit a wide variety of behaviours (Linder, in 1990, gave a detailed description of this approach) or by observing play at the child's own home or within the setting where the existing early intervention programme is carried out.

Fewell et al. (1997) delineate the following advantages of play environment as a setting for the assessment: fewer demands on the child; more choices for the child to demonstrate his or her competencies; more active role of the child in the assessment; play allows the examiner to measure the child's skills across several play tasks and in several domains.

The existing empirical literature indicates that there are numerous benefits to using play assessment and intervention with young children: in fact, the assessment is conducted in the natural environment of play, emphasises learning in the context of daily routine, including child-preferred activities (Buchanan & Johnson, 2009); furthermore, play is motivating and elicits the highest level of a child's functioning (Kelly-Vance, 2008). In comparison to other types of assessment, play-based assessment was found to take less time and resulted in more favourable parent and staff perceptions (Myers et al., 1996); it removes many of the limitations associated with traditional assessment, and in case of children with disabilities, it offers also a number of opportunities to adapt the context to their needs (Fewell et al., 1997).

The *trans-disciplinary play-based assessment* is a method, developed by Linder, that brings together parents and professionals and gives the latter the opportunity to evaluate young children in a natural environment. Trans-disciplinary play-based assessment is a criterion-referenced developmental assessment approach designed to assist the planning of interventions for children with disabilities. During the assessment, the child and his or her parents play with developmentally appropriate toys, while the team members, through observation, assess the child's strengths and weaknesses across all developmental areas. The team members also make observations about the parent–child interaction (King et al., 2009). No specialised test materials are required and the assessment is not standardised: this allows for cross-cultural use. Assessment is unstructured, and a child's developmental status is examined through the informal context of play. The information obtained during the assessment is used to formulate the main goal and objectives of the further individualised intervention.

This type of assessment is less stressful for children and less burdened to the family. Linder (1993) indicates that the advantages of the adoption of such a method include: the use of the natural environment, a better rapport with examiners, parent involvement, major flexibility in testing domains, the assumption of an integrated, holistic perspective on child development, and more useful information for planning intervention. The application of the transdisciplinary play-based assessments needs less time to complete than multidisciplinary standardised assessments (Myers et al., 1996), and it is a cost- and time-effective method (Bergen, 1991).

Bergen (1991) also stresses that developmental levels and delays may be effectively assessed by a team of specialists observing children in a play environment, and that, if the team maintains sensitivity to the elements that should be present for play to occur, the method can be successful without distorting the meaning of play.

14.4 Challenges in Using Play in Early Intervention

The scientific literature sustains the benefits of the play as an integral part in early intervention programmes; nevertheless, there are some challenges and limitations related to the context, parents, and practitioners.

Some early intervention researchers (Bray & Cooper, 2007; Dunst, 2000; Moore, 2008; Rix et al., 2008) report that children with a disability or developmental delay are not always supported to be included in play experiences, and that, play contexts may be overlooked as to their qualities of excellent sites for learning in both centre- or home-based interventions.

In order to achieve the goals of interventions, self-confidence and skills of parents in their abilities to nurture and teach their children must be enhanced (Nwokah et al., 2013). Some studies report parental dissatisfaction with the pressure to carry out activities as part of a programme as well as insufficient support to encourage their child to play (Rix et al., 2008). Matthews and Rix (2013) pointed out as a key challenge for parents involved in early intervention programmes to encourage their child to play and learn through enjoyable, daily childhood experiences. There are specialists complaining that parents do not seem to appreciate the role of play in child development, nor did they prove to be able to play with their children, especially when it comes to shared-object play and pretend play (Cumming & Wong, 2012; Nwokah et al., 2013).

On the other side, some authors (Bray & Cooper, 2007; Moore, 2008; Muir et al., 2008) found that many early childhood practitioners feel unprepared for and lack the knowledge and skills to implement appropriate interventions within their regular play-based programmes and routines. This may create some tensions and may impact the effectiveness of the interventions.

Both specialists and parents of children with disabilities need to be aware of the elements that must be maintained as play activities, as well as about the characteristics that play must assume to be truly playful, to the purpose of maintaining those elements whenever they use play in early intervention (Bergen, 1991).

14.5 Conclusion

Play is a normal activity in the childhood and is widely used in early intervention for children with disabilities. Nevertheless, the overemphasis on using play in early intervention as a means of instruction can be a serious barrier for the development of spontaneous and voluntary play by the child; in addition, in the early intervention, practice play is far from being the only determinant of any learning that takes place (Smith & Gossom, 2010).

Play can contribute significantly in helping children to feel in control with their lives, in using their preferred modes of interaction, and it is also crucial to the development of their self-worth and their competence (Bergen, 1991). The experience of using play in early intervention can contribute for achievement of 'play for the sake of play' for children with disabilities, but to reach this goal, future studies are still needed.

References

Bergen, D. (1987). *Play as a Medium for Learning and Development.* Portsmouth, NH: Heinemann.

Bergen, D. (1991, April). *Play as the Vehicle for Early Intervention with At-Risk Infants and Toddlers.* Paper presented at the Annual Conference of the American Educational Research Association Chicago. Retrieved from: http://files.eric.ed.gov/fulltext/ED335115.pdf.

Blackman, J. A. (2003) Early Intervention: An Overview. In: S. L. Odom, M. J. Hanson, J. A. Blackman, & S. Kaul (Eds.), *Early Intervention Practices around the World.* Baltimore, MD: Paul H. Brookes Publishing.

Bray, P., & Cooper, R. (2007). The play of children with special needs in mainstream and special education settings. *Australian Journal of Early Childhood*, 32(2), 37-42.

Buchanan, M., & Johnson, T. G. (2009). A Second Look at the Play of Young Children with Disabilities. *American Journal of Play*, 2(1), 41-59.

Casby, M. W. (2003). Developmental Assessment of Play: A Model for Early Intervention. *Communication Disorders Quarterly*, 24, 175-183.

Cumming, T., & Wong, S. (2012). Professionals don't play: Challenges for early childhood educators working in a transdisciplinary early intervention team. *Australasian Journal of Early Childhood*, 37(1), 127-135.

Dunst, C. J. (1981). *Infant Learning: A Cognitive-Linguistic Intervention Strategy.* Hingham, MS: Teaching Resources.

Dunst, C. J. (2000). Revisiting "Rethinking early intervention". *Topics in Early Childhood Special Education*, 20, 95-104.

Dunst, C. J. (2007). Early intervention for infants and toddlers with developmental disabilities. In S. L. Odom, R. H. Horner, M. E. Snell, & J. Blacher, J. (Eds.), *Handbook of Developmental Disabilities.* New York, NY: Guilford Press.

Dunst, C. J., & Bruder, M. B. (2002). Valued outcomes of service coordination, early intervention, and natural environments. *Exceptional Children*, 68(3), 361-375.

Fewell, R., Ogura, T., & Wheeden, A. (1997). The Relationship Between Play and Communication Skills in Young Children with Down Syndrome. *Topics in Early Childhood Special Education*, 17(1), 103-118.

Guralnick, M. J. (2001) A Developmental Systems' Model for Early Intervention. *Infants and Young Children*, 14(2), 1-18.

Hanft, B. E., & Pilkington, K. O. (2000). Therapy in natural environments: The means or end goal for early intervention?. *Infants and Young Children*, 12(4), 1-13.

Kasari, C., Gulsrud, A., Freeman, S., Paparella, T, & Hellemann, G (2012). Longitudinal follow up of children with autism receiving targeted interventions on joint attention and play. *Journal of the American Academy of Child and Adolescent Psychiatry*, 51, 487-495.

King, G., Strachan, D., Tucker, M., Duwyn, B., Desserud, S., & Shillington, M. (2009). The Application of a Transdisciplinary Model for Early Intervention Service. *Infants & Young Children*, 22(3), 211-223.

Kelly-Vance, L., & Ryalls, B. O. (2008). Best Practices in Play Assessment and Intervention. *Best Practices in School Psychology V*, 33(2), 549-560.

Lifter, K. (2008). Developmental Play Assessment and Teaching. In J. K. Luiselli, D. C. Russo, & W. P. Christian (Eds.), *Effective Practices for Children with Autism: Educational and Behavioral Support Interventions That Work* (pp. 299-324). New York, NY: Oxford University Press.

Lifter, K., Foster-Sanda, S., Arzamarski, C., Briesch J., & McClure, E. (2011). Overview of Play. Its Uses and Importance in Early Intervention/Early Childhood Special Education. *Infants & Young Children*, 24(3), 225-245.

Linder, T. W. (1990). *Transdisciplinary Play-Based Assessment*. Baltimore, MD: Paul H. Brookes Publishing.

Linder, T. W. (1993). *Transdisciplinary Play-Based Assessment: A Functional Approach to Working with Young Children* (rev. ed.). Baltimore, MD: Paul H. Brookes Publishing.

Matthews A., & Rix, J. (2013). Early intervention: parental involvement, child agency and participation in creative play. *Early Years*, 33(3), 239-251.

Moore, T. (2011). *Early Childhood Intervention Reform Project. Revised Literature Review. Executive Summary*. Department of Education and Early Childhood Development, State of Victoria. Retrieved from: http://www.education.vic.gov.au/Documents/childhood/providers/needs/ecislitreview-execsum.pdf.

Myers, C. L., McBride, S. L., & Peterson, C. A. (1996). Transdisciplinary, play-based assessment in early childhood special education: An examination of social validity. *Topics for Early Childhood Special Education*, 16(1), 102-126.

Muir, K., Tudball, J., & Robinson, S. (2008). *Family Resilience where Families have a Child (0-8) with Disability. Final Report*. Sydney, NSW: Social Policy Research Centre, University of New South Wales.

Nwokah, E., Hsu, H. C., & Gulker, H. (2013). The Use of Play Materials in Early Intervention. The Dilemma of Poverty. *American Journal of Play*, 5 (2), 187-216.

Nwokah, E., & Hope, G. (2006). Emergent Literacy for Children with Special Needs: Developing Positive Interest in Literacy Experiences (Part II). *ACEI: Focus on Infants and Toddlers*, 19, 1-8.

Peeremboom, T. D. (2003). *A literature review of the Treatment and Education for Autistic and related Communication Handicapped Children (TEACCH) program*. Research paper, University of Wisconsin-Stout, Wisconsin, United States of America.

Pierce, D. R. (1997). The Power of Object Play for Infants and Toddlers at Risk for Developmental Delays. In D. L. Parham, & L. S. Fazio (Eds). *Play in Occupational Therapy for Children* (pp. 86-111). St. Louis: Mosby.

Rix, J., Paige-Smith, A., & Jones, H. (2008). 'Until the cows came home': issues for early intervention activities? Parental perspectives on early years learning of their children with Down syndrome. *Contemporary Issues in Early Childhood*, 9(1), 66-79.

Rogers, S. J., & Dawson, G. (2010). *Early Start Denver Model for Young Children with Autism. Promoting Language, Learning, and engagement*. New York and London: Guilford Press.

Sandall, S., Hemmeter, M. L., Smith, B. J., & McLean, M. E. (2005). *DEC Recommended Practices: A Comprehensive Guide for Practical Application*. Missoula, MT: DEC.

Shonkoff, J. P., & Meisels, S. J. (2000). *Handbook of Early Childhood Intervention*. Cambridge, UK: Cambridge University Press.

Smith, P.K., & Gossom, Y. (2010). *Children and Play*. Hoboken, NY: Wiley & Blackwell.

Sutton-Smith, B. (1987). The struggle between sacred play and festive play. In D. Bergen (Ed.), *Play as a Medium for Learning and Development* (pp. 45-48). Portstmouth, MH: Heinemann.

Wolery, M. (2005). DEC recommended practices: Child-focused practices. In S. Sandall, M. L. Hemmeter, B. J. Smith, & M. E. McLean (Eds.), *DEC Recommended Practices: A Comprehensive Guide for Practical Application*. Missoula, MT: DEC.

Odile Perino and Serenella Besio

15 Mainstream Toys for Play

15.1 Introduction

When considering the topic of devices to support the play of children with disabilities, it is important to notice that the contributions may come from two fields: care (rehabilitation, education) and the play itself. Within this second field, play is considered as an activity for pleasure. Its goals and results are not linked with a specific capacity, but concern the child's whole developmental areas: personality, motor, social, cognitive, emotional. Its primary objective—and maybe the only one—is 'to play'.

Pleasure of play, according to Huizinga's definition (1938), comes from free activity; this is the reason for children's autonomy is valued, even if very little, so that they can take charge of their own play and deeply feel themselves, making experience of their own sensitive and emotional being. If it is difficult to share a definition of play, however it is possible to describe playfulness, which is the capacity of any child to fully and freely engage in play, according to Winnicott (1971). Playfulness is represented by four domains: active engagement, internal control, social connection, and joyfulness (Cornelli & Sanderson, 2010).

Toys and games, which belong to the concrete reality around children, are the essential mediators between a child and him or her/self, a child and the others, children, or adults. When used in good conditions, they allow children who have impairments to find playfulness in its four dimensions, in relation to their developmental level.

For this reason, the features of toys and games should be analysed as precisely as possible to find out their specific 'ludic springs' which are suitable for children with disabilities. Moreover, the conditions of access to play materials inside the play areas and the toys' arrangement should also be taken into account, as well as the roles concretely played by adults when supporting children with disabilities as they use toys and games.

The following three milestones belong to the concept of 'play framework' (Perino, 2006), which is a way to think about devices for play in their entirety.

First, concrete objects of play, which are appropriate to the player's abilities and interests, are to be chosen, including all types of games and toys, from rattles to videogames.

Second, the adults' role, parent or professional is to be considered as a major element around the children playing with toys to support free play and feelings of safety and capability. The interpersonal distance between adults and children is modulated according to the physical and psychological needs of the player and the appropriate toys to give playfulness and "the capacity to be alone" (Winnicott,

1958) the opportunity to raise. The adoption of the cited play framework allows adults to adequately separate playtime and play spaces from the other activities, to support children in understanding what are the aims of such moments and why the adults' behaviours change in this specific area and time of life. Adults should always be supportive towards children, encouraging them by positive feedback and congratulating for their achievements.

Third, the physical arrangement of toys and games within play areas is to be minded and verified to the purpose of adjusting it to the players' possibilities. Toys and games can be presented inside thematic areas as isolated or unorganised. Usually, they are shown and kept well in view, except in specific cases. Furthermore, it is important that toys are organised according to their specific possible way of use, to support the child's capacities of classification, seriation, and categorisation, which are at the basis of creating one's own wellbeing (Rosenfeld, 1992).

The theoretical method of choosing toys or games is based on the level of competence required in using them (Garon, 1981; Piaget, 1945). It encompasses the following three steps:

1. To analyse a toy or a game to determine the type of play it subtends or implies, the 'category' it belongs, which depend on its functionalities, without taking too much into account the manufacturer's declared goals. The latter could bring useless elements, for marketing reasons.
2. To detect the physical features of objects, which make them easily usable within their own category: are they big enough, easy to grasp, well-coloured, do they have sounds or not?
3. To verify whether some elements of the objects can make "ludic springs" more attractive than other ones within the same category.

When analysing toys and games, first of all, it is essential to be aware of the toy safety issue (European Parliament and Council, 2009). In many countries, in order to be commercialised, toys must pass safety tests, which mainly concerns the aspects related to their mechanical and physical properties—such as flammability, migration of certain elements (i.e., chemical products), electric systems. Furthermore, age determination is required, when parts of toys are not suitable for children under three years.

If the observance of these standards helps to ensure an overall safety, they do not always guarantee the best security of players:

- Sometimes, children use toys in a way that is not consistent with their intended purposes or proposed age.
- Old or used toys can lose their original qualities to the point that they do not meet anymore the defined safety standard
- Homemade or artisanal toys may not be in line with the safety standards
- Last but not least, in the case of children with disabilities, an increased vigilance is needed because in some cases—due, for example, to sensorial impairments—the use of toys can lead to risky situations

15.2 Devices for the Play of Children with Intellectual Disabilities

Any category of toys can encompass supports of play, depending on the players' interests and levels. The first step to choose appropriate toys is to bear in mind the degree of the players' intellectual impairment and the types of play they would be able to be involved on, consequently choosing toys for practice symbolic, constructive play, or for rules-based games.

Then, within a specific category, the choice depends on the player's interests and tastes for some aesthetic aspects (colours, dimensions, etc.), sensorial effects (texture, smell, etc.), and also for the type of use (action to be made, manipulation, etc.).

Therefore, the choice also depends on the toy's power to facilitate the play activity and to make it particularly attractive to the child.

15.2.1 Toys or Games Features

Practice play. Toys for this type of play provide strong stimuli and require non-complex or few successive actions by the child; each sequence of play is short enough to allow children to keep enjoying play, without losing their interest (which is frequent in young children and in children with intellectual impairment); toys that propose unpredictable effects or with non-visible mechanisms of activation are not useful because they do not give children the opportunity to connect their action with its results, thus maintaining children in a kind of 'magical thinking'. In addition, in order to avoid stereotyped sequences of play and to help the child evolve and adopt new different kinds of gestures and more complex movements, it is useful to provide different objects to make the same ludic activity, for example, pop-up toys that are operated in different ways.

Symbolic play. For a player interested in symbolic play, the shape and size of the toys must be as realistic as possible; moreover, they must represent aspects of the real and daily life environment.

Make-believe play can be difficult for children with intellectual impairments who find it hard to understand that one object can be used as it was another one or that a person can play a different role from his or her own usual one. For many children with intellectual impairments, realistic objects within a thematic area are easier to use for reciprocal exchanges and role recognition, whereas costumes need the support of a reflective metacognitive thought and may be frightening to some of them.

Constructive play. With assembling toys, it is important to pay attention to the duration of play sequences, to avoid lack of interest and maintain the effect of surprise and willingness to continue. When toys are made of parts to be assembled, it is also important to pay attention to the complexity of the connection between them, because in most cases, these children can show difficulties in psychomotor abilities.

Furthermore, it could be hard for them to mentally represent the final result, and consequently, to maintain the attention until it is achieved.

Rule-based play and games. In this case, games must be relevant to the cognitive capacity of the player, particularly regarding reasoning, making hypotheses, deduction, and time of concentration required.

15.2.2 Roles of the Adults

The adults' role is a very important issue to support children with intellectual impairment with finding a form of autonomy in an emotionally secure environment. Adults help children to feel joyfulness in play whilst providing support as patient, enthusiastic partners, and very often, as models during role-play sequences with toys. They can also physically guide the children showing them concretely how to do things, how to use objects. Repetition in learning these practical aspects of play can be useful. Albeit the adults' presence aims to support the child's autonomy, it has been shown that play unfolds on a lower level, without an adult.

Adults should use a gentle, but determined attitude in playing with children, to support them in maintaining their attention, entering a ludic sequence, respect and share the roles and the rules, accept the influence of chance.

15.2.3 Physical Contexts for Play

For children with intellectual impairments, toys for practice play should be as most realistic as possible and should not be displayed as part of a group of toys rather in an isolated way, and shown one after the other, first, to turn on the child's interest and second, to activate exploratory behaviours (Bozena, 2007) and the pleasure of deep understanding. In the case of symbolic play, toys should be proposed inside a consistent play area with complementary objects (for example, a doll and a cradle to play 'mummy', or fruits, dishes and pots to play 'cooking').

15.3 Devices for the Play of Children with Hearing Impairments

When considering free play for children with hearing impairments, the question is: where does joyfulness of play, within the different play categories, come from?

The adults' choice of devices for play depends on the player's interests and tastes concerning a specific type of play activity, a kind of sensorial effect, or the pleasure for a specific kind of manipulations. Therefore, the choice also depends on the physical features of the toys to facilitate the child's play or make it particularly attractive for players with hearing impairments.

Play sequences are less frequent between children and adults when a hearing impairment impedes or makes it difficult to communicate. It is important to encourage play with suitable toys, consistent play areas, and well-informed adults and partners.

15.3.1 Toys or Games Features

Practice play. For all children, the interest towards toys for practice play comes from perceiving the effects of their actions: exploring, understanding cause-and-effect, discovering surprising effects, and enjoying a sense of mastery. At the same time, pleasure of internal control and social connection is there.

In the case of children with hearing impairment, the need to recur to alternative sensorial channels gives importance to toys with visual or tactile stimuli. Visual and tactile effects are especially attractive if they have an immediate significance and if they establish a direct relationship between a cause and an effect.

Symbolic play. As for any child, pleasure of symbolic play is to use things in unusual ways, to be another, express oneself and one's feelings, understand the social environment.

Different toys relative to various topics are required to put various and different roles in place. Realistic toys, in shapes and sizes, are proposed inside thematic areas to suggest complementary roles and support gestural communication. Toys are proposed within consistent ensembles to allow children to go forward in a scenario, for example, a doll and a cradle.

Symbolic play is very important in the case of children with hearing impairment, for it gives them the possibility to explore and use different modes of communication, to act different roles, thus taking the other's point of view and adopting various styles of interaction. The use of verbal language and/or the sign language can introduce interesting variables mainly in this type of play, primarily in the case of social play with peers.

Constructive play. No particular shrewdness is needed for supporting constructive play of children with hearing impairment. Nevertheless, this type of play requires a certain level of concentration on an activity over time, while these children usually do not like to stand and prefer to move around, sometimes without a real scope. This is one of the reasons to choose attractive toys for these children and support them to become concentrated and committed.

Rule-based play and games. The choice is made according to the children's cognitive abilities, and also to the communication abilities needed. The knowledge of the sign language also by the part of the other play companions can be useful in some cases, otherwise solutions should be found to favour communication exchanges, which are adequate to the play rules, so that possible difficulties in reasoning can be overcome too.

15.3.2 Roles of the Adults

As these children might not able to communicate verbally their needs and desires or find it difficult to understand parental and societal rules, they can incur behavioural difficulties. Moreover, hearing parents of deaf children tend to be more directive and controlling in their interactions with their children (Vaccari & Marschark, 1997).

For all these reasons and to facilitate the players' autonomy, the roles of adults, their place, and the distance from children should be very carefully considered.

For example, to sit face-to-face is required to show toys, invite to play as suitable partners, and promote visual or physical interactions. Above all, within a group of children, adults must not forget to ascertain that all the verbal messages are understood by children with hearing impairments. However, when a play sequence between children is starting, adults should not interfere, leaving that communication between them develop as it is possible—through gestures, signs, or verbal cues—so that they can play freely.

15.3.3 Physical Contexts for Play

Toys are always in view, each one is placed inside a specific area according to the type of play they are able to favour.

Symbolic play areas must be organised in a logical and consistent manner for the following reasons:

- To facilitate imitation between children and between children and adults.
- To facilitate adults handing toys, children, as well as gestural and verbal communication.
- To allow children with hearing impairments to observe the other players, to encourage social interactions and joyfulness.
- To allow sharing of complementary roles within the same scenario and the development of that scenario; for example, by installing furniture, so that children play face-to-face instead than side-by-side (Thériault & Doyon, 1987).

15.4 Devices for the Play of Children with Visual Impairments

Where does joyfulness of play, within the different play categories, come from, in the case of children with visual impairments? Of course, also in this case, the choice of devices for play will depend on the player's interests and tastes, but also on the physical features of the toys that will be used.

Furthermore, these devices cannot be considered without regarding consistent play areas and well-informed adults.

15.4.1 Toys or Games Features

Practice play. Pleasure of the first play activities comes from sensorial effects, intellectual motivation in understanding the toys' functions, sense of mastery, and sharing communication about play sequences.

For children with visual impairment, toys must be steady, easy to manipulate with an overall shape, easily understandable by touch. Toys must be made in such a material that can be put inside the mouth for discovering dimensions, shape, and sensorial features. They should also be safe to make it possible an exploration without the eye's control.

Toys for children with visual impairment should give importance to sensorial stimuli other than visual: tactile, hearing, olfactory, kinaesthetic; in the case of sensorimotor play, they must offer diversity, and from time-to-time, unusual sensorial effects (vibration, magnetic effects) so as to arouse curiosity and surprise. They should be activated through precise gestures and offer precise feedback: this will implement children's pleasure and give them eagerness to succeed. Musical toys are particularly attractive when they give immediate and direct feedback to their activation.

Symbolic play. For children play roles as actors, toys must have realistic shapes and must be easy to understand by touch, to facilitate message transmission through objects. Thus, they cannot be too big for the children's hands. When using action figures, for example animals, they must be as realistic as possible to be picked out among others. Anyway, symbolic play should always be introduced by an adult who describes the main theme of play (for example, kitchen, seller, jungle animals, garage) to facilitate entering in a play.

Usually, pretend play is delayed in children with visual impairment with respect to typically developing ones (Lerner et al., 2015); only when they are around 6-9 years old, they will be able to attribute concrete objects a function different from the expected and normal one.

Constructive play. It is useful to propose toys whose elements or parts are not too light in term of weight, to reinforce the sensations of touch and to make the final constructions stand up and in a steady way. Links between these elements should be easy to make, for example, through magnetic or *Velcro* systems; auditory feedback when elements are correctly connected could be useful.

The pieces of puzzles should be well-designed and easily recognisable—better if they are in relief—so that children are willing to complete it; puzzles that are included within borders are preferable as children can better orient their actions and understand by themselves if they have terminated.

Rule-based play and games. Children with visual impairments, as all the other children, usually like to play many games with rules. Of course, in order to find great pleasure in playing and possibly winning boards, pawns and others pieces of the game should be explored by touch, or adapted to this purpose.

The case of colour-blind children should be carefully considered when planning a game with coloured material: some colours are confusing and can make the games hard to play, if not impossible; it is important to be careful with non-differentiated colours and to change them where possible.

What is of utmost importance, nevertheless, is that these children understand well the rules of the game, and above all, that they can 'experience the rule', which organises the players' group around itself. Children with visual impairments can, in this way, experience the value of turn-taking, of decentralising their thoughts from themselves only, by sharing and subjecting to an indisputable rule and also to the chance. In this sense, if the cognitive challenge of the game is lower than expected is not a problem, because the pleasure of practicing the power of the rule is important in itself (Duflos, 1997).

15.4.2 Roles of the Adults

With any category of toys and games, adults help children find their autonomy, even if it has been demonstrated that without adults' assistance, play unfolds at inferior levels. Adults can effectively also act as mediators between children with visual impairments and their companions, so that play can be facilitated, go on, and become joyful and exciting.

For example, in the case of constructive play, frequent feedback on how the construction is going on can be useful because these children find it hard to mentally represent a three-dimensional object to be built as well as the consequent steps to be done for finalising their project. To help children with visual impairments to understand the issues of three-dimensionality and of complex constructions, the best way is to invert the usual phases of constructive play, which are usually made of a building phase and a deconstruction phase (the relative importance of these phases varies depending on the competence and the age of the players). With children with visual impairments, the issue of the third dimension is more difficult, and it must be tested by starting with the second phase. By touching, in fact, the children can realise the size and the volume of the construction already finished. Then, by tearing it down, they come to understand the transition from the complex construction to the simple pieces that compose it. When they truly understand this, they can start to build by adopting a three-dimensional perspective.

15.4.3 Physical Contexts for Play

As children with visual impairments cannot mentally represent the space around them beyond their own body, toys and elements of games must be proposed inside well-demarcated areas to be easy to catch, find, take up again after having been thrown or located in a specific position, and so on. The toys must not 'disappear' far from the players, irrespective to the type of play they belong or to the child's age; auditory feedbacks whenever possible should be used and added.

For pretending play and role-play, toys must be arranged inside thematic areas and consistent ensembles. It is very useful to propose complementary objects on the same theme to support exchange between partners, go forward in the theme, and explore several roles, expressions, and behaviours.

15.5 Devices for the Play of Children with Communication Disorders

When a child has communication disorders, all the types of play can be involved and deprived if not properly and specially prepared and supported. Play is, in fact, made of communication and is communication in itself. Where does joyfulness come from in these cases? Once again, preferences and tastes of the child should be studied, as well as the toys' features and the play context organisation.

15.5.1 Toys or Games Features

Practice play. Usually, children with communication disorders like very much to enjoy body movement play and are interested in toys that facilitate and intensify these kinds of play. Consequently, they would like toys that support gross motor skills, like balls, slides, and all the devices that can be found at the playground. According to Fontaine (2005), communication between children is intense and implemented during play on structures for gross motors skills than with small toys.

Symbolic play. Children with communications disorders do not like at all to experience situations in which their difficulties can be reveiled to their playmates, and consequently, highlighted. Thus, during role-playing, they do not act as protagonists, but prefer to be 'followers'. On the other hand, they need to express their emotions and find the right words or modes to tell the world how they feel. While pretending play can give them the possibility to enlarge and sustain their knowledge of the semantic field of words, including its metaphorical aspects, playing roles can be interesting for letting them to imagine themselves in situations and roles different from the usual ones, thus understanding and using new words, new concepts, new ways of communicating: this is the case of acting in roles and also useful for them; puppets, puppetry, disguises, figures, toys based on cartoons, play dough, etc.

When these children use systems of Alternative Augmentative Communication (AAC), adaptations should be made to toys and play contexts to give them the possibility to take part actively to the play situation.

Constructive play. Usually, there is no specific attention to adopt to constructive play in the case of children with communication disorders.

Rule-based play and games. This type of play should usually be easy to play, depending on the intellectual level of the players. The main goal is to support children to have the possibility to win this type of games, as they are often losers with them; thus, the role of chance should be taken into consideration, and whenever possible, controlled. Obviously, to support play for the sake of play, the games must not be directly addressed to the precise children's deficit.

It is important also to have some parts of the board games translated into written words or into symbols if the child uses AAC codes.

15.5.2 Roles of the Adults

The main role of adults, when they act as playmates of children with communication disorders, is to add language to all the play sequences, to let them better understand the play rules, to support them in expressing their feelings and ideas, as well as to facilitate the play relationships, by decoding their peers' proposals and also by letting peers understanding their modalities of communication. Depending on the type of impairment, verbal language can be accompanied by gestures, or written words or symbols.

15.5.3 Physical Contexts for Play

Toys are installed inside specific areas of the environment where play activities will take place. A role-play area is installed to enable children to play face-to-face, to support communication, and to facilitate complementary roles. Many devices and materials are prepared and made available as a support for AAC users; they can be created on the basis of the play activity or of a player's specific communication needs, or made available as general-purpose support tools. In some cases, typical functioning children should be introduced to the knowledge and use of these particular communication modes.

15.6 Devices for the Play of Children with Physical Impairments

As for any other child, also for children with physical impairments joyfulness of play comes from the satisfaction of the player's interest and tastes. Therefore, the choice of toys depends on their physical features, and the identification of the play activity is related to the specific preferences of the child as well as on his or her abilities and competences. Due to their difficulties in movement, which often show up as slowness, fatigue, and inaccuracy, time of play activities and sequences is one of the most important issues to be addressed.

It should not been forgotten that physical impairments are often associated with other kinds of impairments, such as language and communication disorders, intellectual and/or sensorial impairments. In these cases, the access to play activities becomes even more difficult and complex.

15.6.1 Toys or Games Features

All the toys' categories can be proposed to children with physical impairments, but it is essential to take into account first the movements that are necessary to use the toys; it should be considered; in particular:

a. how the toy can be used: with which parts of the body, if it is possible to use it by means of other parts of the body;
b. which kinds of action are needed (grasping, pulling, pushing, inserting, plugging, sliding, picking up, combining, and so on);
c. which precision and coordination of movements are required and also to what extent strength should be adopted.

Modification to traditional and mainstream toys should be considered by substituting the activation systems, introducing handles, buttons, grasping solutions, and other possible devices, so that the toy can be easier used by the child; these modifications are, of course, different from child to child, because they are created or adopted on his or her own movement abilities. More complex modifications—due in more complex movement impairments—very often include the use of a personal computer as a mean to control concrete objects on the environment.

Second, often children with physical impairments have less perseverance in play situation as well as in other daily activities due to the difficulties they meet and the time they require to complete a task: for this reason, short play sessions are preferable, so that they can maintain their interest and commitment.

Third, it is not infrequent that these children are sitting in wheelchairs or use other supports, and this fact should be taken into account also to choose toys and play activities: a wheelchair imposes some distance from the floor, for example, or requires a suitable height of tables or other work surfaces, so that they can have a complete visual control on the toy or game and can easily reach and use them as they want.

Practice play. Toys for this type of play are solid, easy to hold and to be used, steady for sensorimotor and gross motor skills play. They are of good quality for lighting, musical, tactile, and other effects. The ludic springs are well-defined and easy-to-produce even if physical possibilities are reduced in terms of strength and gestural precision. The use of these toys should also be carefully considered in relation to the children's motor devices to facilitate play and make it as safe as possible.

Outdoors play activities should also be included, because kinaesthetic discovering is important to create awareness of one's own body as a whole.

Symbolic play. Toys are realistic and easy to use; they allow children to take on roles and enter situations to experiment in play what they cannot do and live in their real life. Symbolic play is the way for children with physical impairments to express their emotional life, fears, dreams, and satisfactions. Dolls and other traditional toys for symbolic play (puppets, theatre characters, miniature objects, etc.) can be chosen or modified for being easy to use. Costumes and disguises should also include wheelchairs and other movement supports to give these children the possibility to fully take part in play sessions together with their peers.

Constructive play. To allow these children to play with construction toys, it is essential to choose them according to the size of pieces and their weight, nor too small nor too heavy. The most important is to consider carefully the mechanism to assemble the elements; magnetic or *Velcro* links are preferable, so that construction play becomes possible even in case of imprecise gestures or jerky movements. In some cases, mainstream toys can be modified, so that they can be manipulated and used: handles and various kinds of systems to take the pieces and assemble or disassemble them can be adopted.

Rule-based play and games. When rule-based play is based on movement, only seldom it is proposed to these children, due to their physical impairment, even if they can take place in the game by playing different roles within the game; some specific types of games have been invented—the most famous one is 'baskin'—and are currently being disseminated. Board games can be difficult to play due to their form and dimension, but also in this case, some changes can be undertaken to enlarge the accessibility of the material. Pawns are easy to grasp with sometimes magnetic bases, while bigger dice are easy to throw and control or can be replaced with other devices.

Play time is shortened when possible, mainly for decreasing the fatigue due to a prolonged motor engagement; in fact, tiredness related to difficulties in controlling movements may adversely affect the motivation and the quality of the involvement in the game.

15.6.2 Roles of the Adults

Children with physical impairments are more dependent on the others' supports in their life, and this is what happens also in playing. As play companions, adults should let them take their time, without taking their place; they should wait for children to play and have the opportunity to give their autonomous suggestions to go on in playing, for example, by transforming toy functions or game rules.

The adults' role is also to become an effective play mediator, so that these children's peers can be supported in creating fruitful and joyful interactions; sometimes, only some tricks are needed to let play activities start and go on in a satisfactory way. When other kinds of impairments are associated to the physical one, the role of the adults can be even more relevant, as they have to help peers in interpreting, communicating, acting as facilitators or scaffolders in the best way.

15.6.3 Physical Contexts of Playing

Toys and games are carefully selected, according to an analysis of their components; toys in many cases should be modified and made accessible.

Space is one of the most important aspects of the play context in this case: play environments should be large enough to facilitate children's movement, to let them move autonomously; their use of motor devices should be carefully considered, both as to space dimensions and as to the height and accessibility of work surfaces.

Furthermore, appropriate and comfortable play situations should be prepared, as a child sitting in a wheelchair can be in a higher or lower position with respect to his or her peers, and, according to the type of play, this may require the adoption of certain logistic measures, so that gazes can be exchanged, the materials for playing can be available, and so on.

15.7 Devices for the Play of Children with Autism Spectrum Disorders

Any category of play can encompass supports of play, depending on the players' interests and developmental levels. For children with ASD, the type and degree of impairment—which explicitly matter human relationships, symbolic functions, and play development—can vary widely. Furthermore, intellectual disability can be associated to other impairments, as well as specific extraordinary abilities—the so-called 'islets of abilities' or 'splinter skills'.

All these aspects should be considered before proposing toys or games to these children, who in some cases, actually do not seem to enjoy play or wish to be involved in.

15.7.1 Toys or Games Features

Within all toys' or games' categories, objects may not be replaced every day. For the players' emotional wellbeing, a balance has to be found between well-known toys and games, and new ones. In order to get a kind of continuity and logical evolution within the play activities, choice of toys and games varies from already known functionalities to different ones: this is to make sure that games have common traits with functions that evolve from one to the other.

Practice play. In most cases, play with objects consists of two steps: the first consists of an exploration of the overall shape of objects without paying attention to their use, while only later an understanding of the functionalities of these objects takes place.

Children with ASD are not attracted by the overall shape of the objects, as they are more interested by some specific aspects, or small details. When proposing toys to attract their attention, weight is an interesting element due to proprioceptive sensations and the body consciousness; texture of the object is also important, as well as sensorial feedback it can produce (visual—mainly light—auditory). Sometimes, this feedback is only provoked by the particular way adopted by the child in using the toy. The cause-and-effect relationship is also a positive element of toys for children with ASD, if it is easy to perceive and understand.

Some toys for practice play are particularly interesting as they can initiate social connection, for example, by throwing, catching, giving, and giving back.

Symbolic play. Role-playing is particularly tricky for these children who often feel challenged by representing and changing roles, adopting the point of view of other persons, acting as if they were other persons.

This play activity is then initiated by adults who help in simplifying roles and activities and break it down into subsequent steps, each of them corresponding to one specific isolated action with objects (for example, interpreting 'being a musician' only by playing drums).

For symbolic play with figurines and miniatures, isolated toys are more appropriate than ensembles to support a precise play activity: for example, playing with a car and moving it forward instead of managing a whole garage. Once effective play sessions with one object are obtained, it becomes possible to use toys that can be related to the same topic to expand the children's play.

Constructive play. For children with ASD, adults propose games that have a clear goal and end; they encourage players by showing them what it is possible to do with this type of toys, and how. They choose the toys that can be used for a short play time, so that children finish the activity quickly and feel successful.

Assembling games are changed from time to time to make play evolve according to the different types of connections between the elements. In some cases, children with ASD can become and reveal experts in those types of toys and spend a lot of time in assembling small elements not always according to a clear and recognisable project of construction. Putting together pieces, completing a puzzle as quickly as possible, repeating for the sake of repetition may seem, in these cases, the only scope of their play. More complex toys in these cases can be proposed to interrupt the sterile repetition of gestures and activities, if this reiteration is perceived as devoid of joy.

Rule-based play and games. Very often, rules are simplified and games shortened for these children, while instructions are made as clear as possible. Games that are more appreciated by children with ASD are association games where the ludic spring is given by activities of comparison and differentiation.

Children with ASD need simple rules because the social situation is so challenging for them that it is essential that rules are very easy to understand for playing with joyfulness. Rules can be contemporarily a problem and an advantage for children with ASD: in fact, they facilitate understanding of the play activity, because they put clear limits to control the situation; on the other hand, they highlight the tendency of these children to act in a well-regulated and repetitive manner and they prevent them from the adoption of flexible shortcuts during the activity. Then, there is the possibility that they appreciate this type of toys and games; this could be a way, for them, to face human relationships.

15.7.2 Roles of the Adults

Adults whom the children know well are essential, so that they are not frightened by the social context. Adults should act as play partners or models, and usually, they propose the play sequences.

They can initiate role-playing and encourage it by reminding the children stories and tales they already know and proposing to interpret them. In the case of construction play, the adults show examples of how to continue the construction and avoid the children with ASD to repeat always the same sequence—for example, asking them to do something new, or to do it in a different way—or propose the children to explain which is their project.

In rule-based games, one of the roles of adults is to simplify the play situation to avoid or minimise frustrations; for example, within games such as snakes and ladders, by taking the dice off so that each player's turn is respected (Hogan, 1997).

15.7.3 Physical Contexts for Play

For emotional comfort and wellbeing, the number of toys presented at the same time is reduced to two or three, and the overall environment is quiet, without sudden noise or changes in lighting. As social relations with non-familiar people are not easy for these children, adults promote parallel play between players by putting in place more thematic play areas and supporting children with ASD, so that they can imitate and play on their own, but alongside other children.

15.8 Devices for the Play of Children with Multiple Disabilities

To support children with multiple disabilities in play, adults use to present toys or mainstream objects as supports of play, depending on the players' levels, interests, and tastes. Play is an activity that involves the child's whole personality: emotional, intellectual, social, physical. The free play and the autonomy of the player remain concepts that keep their meaning irrespective to the importance of disability. It is the reason why play is so important for children with multiple disabilities.

As multiple disabilities always concern sensorial impairment, often the focus of the play activity is on sensorimotor toys to support the sensorial and kinaesthetic experiences; it is anyway possible to propose also toys related to other types of play, mainly with the support of an adult.

With respect to the type of impairments these children have, possible additional supports can be considered: for example, the need to adopt codes of AAC, to recur to specialised materials and toys or to on-purpose modification of mainstream toys, to choose toys that can offer precise sensorial stimuli, and so on.

15.8.1 Toys or Games Features

Practice play. Toys for play are chosen on the basis of the child's possibilities to explore them; objects that can offer multisensorial and rich proprioceptive experience should be preferred. Smaller toys are proposed where sensorial stimuli they offer are identifiable and rely on proprioceptive sensorial abilities, such as vibration.

Symbolic play. Depending on the players' capabilities, role-play sequences can be developed, mainly with realistic toys or miniature, as they help to play precise roles and to represent specific real situations.

Constructive play. The presence of a possible visual impairment introduces many limits and constraints to the type of toys that can be used for constructive play; furthermore, the possibility to develop a project and to mentally represent the final result of a construction can be reduced, mainly due to multiple sensorial impairments. Thus, careful attention should be dedicated during the selection phase, as to the tactile and auditory aspects of the toys. Sizeable toys with assembling systems must be easy to use without requiring strength.

Rule-based play and games. They should be consistent with the players' competences, their ability to concentrate, and their interests. With respect to the different types of sensorial impairments that are involved in the multiple disability, adapted or alternative board games can be used, which recur to special communication systems or to specific devices.

15.8.2 Roles of the Adults

Adults must be convinced that play is essential for children with multiple disabilities too. A kind of empathy is necessary, with verbalisation of what is going to happen, using physical contacts, for example. Explaining, giving meaning, encouraging, congratulating, and being a patient and delighted partner are the main roles of adults in play with children with multiple disabilities. They also should pay attention to give children enough time to play.

15.8.3 Physical Contexts of Play

The physical context in these cases should be particularly studied and arranged to avoid any risk of injury, and at the same time, to motivate children with multiple disabilities to engage in play activities even if they can at first appear noisy, disturbing, and challenging.

According to the different types of sensorial impairments that are present, the context should be well-defined, protected, sometimes with clear and identifiable boundaries. In some cases, the room itself becomes a play occasion or object, as sensorial stimuli can be offered by the floor, or the ceiling. To maintain interest in play, it is essential to regularly change toys and games while maintaining the same or nearly the same ludic springs.

In a socially inclusive context, within a free play sequence, it is possible to make children with multiple disabilities meet typically developing peers, on a condition that play areas are organised with a sensorial quiet atmosphere for what concerns 'sensorial proximity', sensorial contacts, and ludic relationships (Hulsegge & Verheul, 1989).

15.9 Conclusion

The action of playing can be defined as a subtle alchemy brought about by the coming together of a subject, an object, circumstances, and others subjects. The relationship between a human being and his or her environment is always or most always organised around a material element, a sensorial and cognitive artefact that leads to make activities. Paradoxically, this relationship is at the core of what makes a human's thinking independent from our abilities, competences, or age.

Every human action is guided by the interaction with a physical element; playing, which in essence is an activity, needs a mediating object to allow the child to express himself or herself.

While playing, the inclusion of children with disabilities is achieved by providing them with mainstream toys selected according to their capacities: first, to play with others and second, to help parents to give the childhood more importance than to the disability.

Unfortunately, the complexity of toys, depending on their cultural and market aspects, and on what they represent from one generation to the next leads adults to consider them as inadequate for the capacities of children with disabilities. It is, hence, essential to provide mainstream adequate toys accompanied by empathic helpers who are able to facilitate the utmost important interactions between the player and a toy, so that the player's interest can be triggered.

Toys are the first thing adults have in mind when they think to give a child a very appreciated present, or simply a tool to play. But, toys are never neutral, and there is not a toy that suits everyone; differences related to the chronological age, to personal attitudes, to gender, to familiar and cultural traditions, to various ways of life should be considered when choosing a toy. There are toys for indoor and for outdoor spaces, for playing alone or with the peers or even with the adults, for playing together or for winning over the others, and there are toys that favour different types of play, as this chapter has tried to demonstrate. Furthermore, the world around the child is full of objects that can become toys, depending on the curiosity, the imagination, the situation, the play companions.

Nevertheless, there are some other characteristics that should be taken into serious consideration, especially when the child who receives or is offered the toy has some kind of impairment: its usability and accessibility. Does it meet the child's possibilities to interact with it, to enjoy it? Does it respond to the child's preferences and abilities? Does it help the child to overcome his or her difficulties or limitations, or on the contrary does it pose additional limitations? Does it create discouragement because it is difficult or impossible to be used by the child or because it is too simple in comparison with the child's possibilities and expectations? Is it attractive enough to potentially augment the opportunity to play with friends? Is it challenging enough to give the child the opportunity to explore new, more complex types of play?

Adults—parents, teachers, professionals—might need advice when choosing the right toy for these children; they should be accompanied to merge in the most fruitful way the child's and the toy's characteristics in the perspective of creating the best opportunity to have fun and to fully enjoy play. They also would know more about how to play with these children, how to support motivation and engagement even when tiredness, fatigue, indifference, or frustration come forward, and also how to create the more promising contexts for playing, especially inclusive ones.

The chapter has presented some hints on this topic, and should be considered, in the authors' intentions, as a path to make the first steps, to proceed then towards more complex and exhaustive routes in the near future.

References

Albaret, J. M., & Zanone, P. G. (2000). Une approche dynamique du trouble d'acquisition de la coordination. Evolutions Psychomotrices, *Approche Neurologique des Apprentissages chez l'Enfant*, 12(59), 126-136.

Aufauvre, M. R. (1980). *Apprendre à jouer, apprendre à vivre* [Learning to play, learning to live]. Paris, F: Delachaux et Niestlé.

Barker, D. H., Quittner, A. L., Fink, N. E., & Eisenberg, L. S. (2009). Predicting behavior problems in deaf and hearing children: The influences of language, attention, and parent–child communication, *Developmental Psychopathology*, 21(2), 373-392.

Bozena, M. (2007). *Exploratory Play and Cognitive Activity, Several Perspectives on Children's Play*. Antwerp, B: Garant.

Bruner, J. (1991). *Le développement de l'enfant, savoir-faire, savoir dire* [Child development, knowing to do, knowing to say], Paris, F: Puf.

Caffari-Viallon, R. (1988). *Pour que les enfants jouent* [Let the children play]. Lausanne, CH: EESP.

Château, J. (1985). *L'enfant et le jeu* [Child and play]. Paris, F: éditions Du Scarabée.

Cornelli, S., & Sanderson, R. (2010). *Towards a New Measure of Playfulness: The Capacity to Fully and Freely Engage in Play*. Chicago, IL, Loyola University. Retrieved from: http://ecommons.luc.edu/luc_diss/232.

Csíkszentmihályi, M. (1990). *Flow: the Psychology of Optimal experience*. New York, NY: Harper & Row.

Delaye, L., Dufour, S., Perino, O., & Sanches, C. (2007). *Guide Handilud*. Lyon, F: FM2J-ed.

Duflos, C. (1997). *Jouer et philosopher* [To play and to philosophise]. Paris, F: Presses Universitaires de France.

European Parliament and Council (2009). Directive 2009/48/EC on the Safety of Toys. *Official Journal of the European Union*, June the 18th.

Fontaine, A. M. (2005). Écologie développementale des premières interactions entre enfants: effet des matériels de jeu [Developmental ecology of the first interaction among children: effects of the play materials]. *Enfance*, 2(57), 137-154.

Garon, D. (2002). *Le Système ESAR*. Québec, CDN: Le cercle de la librairie.

Garvey, C. (1990). *Play*. Cambridge, MA: Harvard University Press.

Gillet, P. (2013). *Neuropsychologie de l'autisme chez l'enfant* [Neuropsychology of autism in childhood]. Bruxelles, B: De Boeck Solal.

Goleman, D. (1997). *L'intelligence émotionnelle* [Emotional intelligence]. Paris, F: R. Laffont.

Gutton, P. (1972). *Le jeu de l'enfant* [The play of the child]. Paris, F: Larousse université.

Hogan, K. (1997). *Non Verbal Thinking, Communication, Imitation, and Play Skills from a Developmental Perspective*. Chapel Hill, NC: North Carolina University, division TEACCH.

Huizinga, J. (1955). *Homo Ludens, essai sur la fonction sociale du jeu*. Paris, F: Gallimard.

Hulsegge, J., & Verheul, A. (1989). *Snoezelen, un autre monde* [Snoezelen, another world]. Namur (B): Editions Erasme.

Jambor, T., & Van Gils, J. (2007). *Several Perspectives on Children's Play*. Antwerp, B: Garant.

Lerner, R. M., Liben, L. S., & Mueller, U. (2015). *Handbook of Child Psychology and Developmental Science, Volume 2, Cognitive Processes, 7th Edition*. New York, NY: Wiley.

Ludoscopes (1996-2009). *Sélections annuelles de jeux et jouets analysés et commentés* [Annual selections of play and toys analysis and reviews]. Lyon, F: Ass Quai des Ludes.

Michelet, A. (1972). *Les outils de l'enfance T. 1 et 2* [The tools of childhood]. Paris, F: Delachaux et Niestlé.

Perino, O. et al.. (2011). *C.O.L. Classement des objets ludiques* [A classification of ludic objects]. Lyon, F: FM2J-ed.

Perino, O. (2014). *Des espaces pour jouer, pourquoi les concevoir et comment les analyser* [Spaces for playing, why to design them and how to analyse them]. Toulouse, F: Eres éditions.
Piaget, J. (1945). *La formation du symbole chez l'enfant* [Play, dreams and imitation in childhood]. Neuchatel, CH: Delachaux et Niestlé.
Premack, D., & Premack, A. (2003). *Le bébé, le singe et l'homme* [Child, ape and man]. Paris, F: Odile Jacob.
Rosenfeld, I. (1992). *La conscience activité principale du cerveau* [Consciousness, principal activity of the brain]. Paris, F: Flammarion.
Schoggen, P. (1989). *Behavior Settings: A Revision and extension of Roger G. Barker's Ecological Psychology*. Stanford, CA: Stanford University Press.
Skalická, M. (2000). *How Can We Support Visual Functioning of Young Children with Multiple Impairment?* Cracow: International Council for Education of People with Visual Impairment. Retrieved from: http://www.icevi-europe.org/cracow2000/proceedings/index.html.
Stambak, M., & Sinclair, H. (1990). *Les jeux de fiction entre enfants de 3 ans* [Pretend play in three-year-old children]. Paris, F: Presses Universitaires de France.
Thierault, J., & Doyon, M. (1987). *Projet d'analyse du matériel éducatif des classes maternelles* [A project to analyse educational materials at the kindergarten]. Québec, CDN: Université de Chicoutimi.
Vaccari, C., & Marschark, M. (1997). Communication between parents and deaf children: implications for social-emotional development. *The Journal of Child Psychology, Psychiatry*, 38(7), 793-801.
Vygotskij, L. S. (2002). Play and its role in the mental development of the child. *Psychology and Marxism*, internet archive [1933].
Vygotskij, L. S., & Cole, M. (1978). *Mind in Society. The Development of Higher Psychological Processes*. Cambridge, MA: Harvard University Press.
Winnicott, D. W. (1958). The Capacity to be Alone. *International Journal Psycho-Analysis*, 39, 416-420.
Winnicott, D. W. (1975). *Jeu et réalité* [Play and reality]. Paris, F: Gallimard.

Angharad Beckett, Carol Barron, Nan Cannon Jones, Marieke Coussens, Annemie Desoete, Helen Lynch, Maria Prellwitz, and Deborah Fenney Salkeld

16 Influence of Environmental Factors on Play for Children with Disabilities – An Overview

16.1 Introduction

This chapter considers the impact of the environment on the play experience of disabled children or children with disabilities. The International Classification of Functioning (ICF) defines 'environment' as "social attitudes, architectural features, legal and social structures, as well as climate, terrain and so forth" (WHO 2002:10). Whilst this is a helpful opening definition of 'environment', for the purpose of this chapter, we adopt the following *elaboration* of the concept of social environment, which, we argue, is in keeping with the WHO's definition:

> "the immediate physical surroundings, social relationships, and cultural milieus within which defined groups of people function and interact. Components (...) include built infrastructure; (...) social and economic processes; wealth; social, human, and health services; power relations; government; (...) social inequality; cultural practices; the arts; religious institutions and practices; and beliefs about place and community. The social environment subsumes many aspects of the physical environment, given that contemporary landscapes (...) and other natural resources have been at least partially configured by human social processes" (Barnett & Casper, 2001:465).

As stated in the preamble to the United Nation Convention on the Rights of Persons with Disabilities (UNCRPD, 2007, para. e), disability 'results from the interaction between persons with impairments and attitudinal and environmental barriers that hinder their full and effective participation in society on an equal basis with others'. Whilst the language of the UNCRPD may differ slightly from that of the ICF, the ICF model shares this understanding of disability. Environmental factors are understood to operate as barriers or facilitators of people with disabilities; to be *enabling* or *constraining*.

In this chapter, we focus on the constraining—or *disabling*—aspects of the environment on the play experiences and opportunities of children with disabilities. This is not because we fail to recognise that there are examples of good practice 'out there', where children with disabilities have been empowered in their play. Such examples exist and are to be celebrated. They are, however, the exception rather than the rule.

Taking the UK as an example, the findings of a recent UK Public Inquiry by the Charity Sense, chaired by Lord Blunkett and Lesley Rogers, are revealing. The inquiry exposed many environmental factors acting as barriers to play for children with multiple disabilities. The inquiry found that amongst parents of children with disabilities interviewed, 81% reported difficulties in accessing the mainstream play groups and local play opportunities for their child. Many said that they had experienced negative attitudes towards their child, and that this was the most significant barrier to accessing the mainstream play settings. Fifty-one percent of the parents said their child had been intentionally excluded from play opportunities by providers of play. Forty percent said that they faced additional financial costs when seeking to access play opportunities. Many of the families consulted said there was a lack of specialist support that could be accessed locally and were having to make long journeys to access play settings. The inquiry also found that: many play settings were not accessible to children with multiple needs; few settings had been designed to welcome and support parents and non-disabled siblings, so that they could play together with a child with disabilities; levels of awareness and relevant training in medical conditions, communication methods, and multiple disabilities by play professionals act as barriers to children accessing play provision; misguided notions of 'health and safety' can result in children with disabilities, sometimes being denied the right to play (Sense, 2016). Further, in June 2016, the advanced, unedited version of the UNCRC Committee on the Rights of the Child's 'Concluding observations on the fifth periodic report of the United Kingdom of Great Britain and Northern Ireland' highlighted insufficient places and facilities for play and leisure for children in the UK, *in particular those accessible for children with disabilities* (our emphasis). We suspect that the situation in the UK would resonate with many countries across Europe and beyond.

Our emphasis on barriers—*disabling* barriers—is a reflection of our adoption within this chapter of perspectives from interdisciplinary Disability Studies. Disability Studies have challenged the traditional approaches to childhood disability. In 1998, a leading author in this field, Mark Priestley, proposed an agenda for research in this area. Research at that time, he argued, had become "preoccupied with impairment, vulnerability and service usage" and needed to recognise children with disabilities as "social actors, negotiating complex identities within a *disabling environment*" (Priestley, 1998:207, our emphasis). Research, he stated, needed to be informed by new Disability Studies approaches to understanding disability. This new approach represented a sustained critique of the 'individual model' of disability (Oliver, 1990) and versions of this—that is, 'medical' and 'personal tragedy' models—which view disability as a personal predicament. Whilst not denying the existence or impact of impairments, this approach, which has come to characterise the approach taken by many/most academics in Disability Studies, considers the 'problem' of disability to reside within society, not within individual minds or bodies. From a Disability Studies perspective, disability is a form of social oppression, not simply restricted activity (however, caused) and results from actions on the part of the non-disabled majority. These actions—through social structures, organisations, professional practice, and interpersonal interaction—impact negatively on the lives of people with disabilities. Disability is a social relational category—an effect and quality of relationships of power and exclusion between groups in our societies (Thomas, 2004). This approach, thus, involved a paradigm shift. Disability became understood as a *social* rather than an individual pathology (Goodley, 2014); a public issue, not simply a personal trouble (Borsay, 1986).

Allied as it is to the disabled people's movement and their politicisation of 'disability', Disability Studies have long worked to expose environmental factors that act as barriers in the lives of people with disabilities, seeing this as the first step towards challenging and dismantling these barriers. In this chapter, we take such an approach. We identify a range of environmental barriers that 'disable' play for children with disabilities, and by doing so, propose avenues for developing enabling play environments for these children. Although in practice, many of these barriers are inter-related, for the purposes of this chapter, we distinguish different broad barrier types—physical, social, political, and cultural—occurring in a selection of social situations or *locations*—built environment, educational settings, home, and natural environments. These locations can also overlap (e.g., in the case of home schooling or nature playgrounds in school settings). We distinguish them only to point to issues that may be experienced differently in particular locations and to suggest specific avenues for further research.

16.2 Barriers to Play for Children with Disabilities within Four Key Contexts

General Comment 17 on the UNCRC stresses that children with disabilities encounter 'multiple barriers' in relation to the rights provided in Article 31, including exclusion from social situations, where play takes place and friendships can be formed, isolation, cultural attitudes, and stereotypes, physical inaccessibility, and exclusionary or ineffective policies. Before considering some of these barriers manifesting within our four key location types, we highlight the importance of certain political and cultural barriers impacting *across* these locations. First, political barriers: play for children with disabilities is not always given sufficient attention by policy makers. At a global level, both the UNCRC (Article 31) and the UNCRPD (Article 30) enshrine the right of children with disabilities to play and leisure or recreation. Two General Comments on articles of the UNCRC, however, have highlighted the key difficulties in protecting and upholding these rights. In Europe, despite universal ratification of the UNCRC, different states have progressed at different rates with regard to acknowledging and properly resourcing play provision for children with disabilities (Barron et al., *forthcoming*). There is a slippage between the ambitions set out within the international conventions and their operation in relation to national legislation, policy, and practice. Further research needs to establish how different states in Europe are developing policies promoting inclusive play and monitoring their effectiveness.

In terms of cultural barriers, although studies indicate that children with disabilities enjoy similar activities to their non-disabled peers (Engel-Yeger et al., 2009; Hilton et al., 2008; Imms et al., 2008), play is often positioned or understood differently for them. Problematic discourses of play exist and have *real effects* (Joseph & Roberts, 2007) in terms of the exclusion of children with disabilities. These children are more likely to be considered 'deficient' in the abilities necessary for play, and consequently, to be subject to greater adult intervention and surveillance in their play activities, reducing their opportunities for free play (Goodley & Runswick-Cole, 2010). Their play, as for many children, but perhaps more acutely in the case of children with disabilities, is also more likely to be subject to the "play as progress" rhetoric, which involves the "subordination of intrinsic play functions to other extrinsic developmental functions" (Sutton-Smith, 1997: 18). This means that children with disabilities risk missing out on experiencing play for its own sake and its associated benefits.

We now turn to additional and specific barriers identified within our four key locations. In what follows, we draw upon a narrative review of the existing international research into barriers to play for children with disabilities undertaken by the authors for the LUDI network and which is considered in depth within Barron et al. (*forthcoming*).

16.2.1 Barriers in the Built Environment

A 'built environment' refers to the human-made space in which a human activity takes place. For children playing, such spaces might include playgrounds, parks, and other community play spaces. The outdoor public playground (Moore & Lynch, 2015; Webb, 2003) has been the main focus of research into play for children with disabilities within built environments. Evidence suggests that these children encounter physical barriers and are less playful where there is inadequate design—that is, when those designing and providing play spaces have insufficient knowledge about disability and universal design (Dunn & Moore, 2005; Prellwitz & Tamm, 1999; Rigby & Gaik, 2007; Woolley, 2013). Physical access to play spaces is an essential prerequisite to play for children with disabilities.

The absence of or inaccessibility of play resources or materials is also important, as are other issues that may create barriers within play spaces: noise, over-crowding, temperature, unsuitable lighting, design, inaccessible surfaces, etc., depending on the needs of individual children (Law et al., 1999; Rimmer et al., 2004). Finding solutions to these barriers can be challenging, however, because 'special' accessible features in playgrounds (as opposed to fully integrated accessibility) can also lead to segregation (Dunn & Moore, 2005).

Inaccessible built environments and the resulting lack of interaction between children with and without disabilities can reinforce attitudinal barriers (Atmakur, 2013). Exclusion of children with disabilities by non-disabled peers within this type of location (e.g., playgrounds) is as yet under-researched, but on the basis of existing evidence about children's experiences of play in a variety of contexts, this is likely to be a significant problem. Children with disabilities have reported that they are not asked to play by other children or that they have been told that they are not welcome to join in games (Spencer-Cavaliere & Watkinson, 2010). Children with disabilities may also self-exclude through fear of being seen to use play equipment in the 'wrong way', and so, wait until playgrounds are empty before using it (Prellwitz & Skar, 2007). Alternatively, it may be necessary for parents to be present in play situations, for example, to provide assistance to move around and use playground equipment where the design of the playground does not support the child's independent mobility (Prellwitz & Skar, 2007). Children have indicated that they would prefer to use playgrounds independently. Parental anxieties about stigma felt by their children in such situations has led some families to avoid playgrounds (Prellwitz, 2007).

16.2.2 Barriers in Educational Settings

Educational settings may be formal (e.g., kindergarten, primary and secondary school classrooms) or informal (e.g., school playgrounds and after-school clubs). Such settings should provide a safe environment for children's development, foster active learning, and encourage positive peer relations (Moyles, 2013).

Evidence suggests that physical barriers exist within school buildings in some countries (Santer et al., 2007), reflecting the historic exclusion of children with disabilities from education, or from 'mainstream' education. Accessibility for these children within school playgrounds is not always considered (Rigby & Gaik, 2007), leading them to encounter similar difficulties to those in other outdoor play settings (as aforementioned). Attitudinal barriers are also present within this type of environment. Exclusion by peers has been reported by children with disabilities and can occur during recess, for example (Spencer-Cavaliere & Watkinson, 2010; Taub & Greer, 2000).

One way educational settings differ from wider built or natural environment settings is that teachers and other education professionals are often present. Evidence suggests that the attitude and behaviour of teachers can play a significant role in relation to play for children with disabilities. Teachers initiate and facilitate play between children with and without disabilities through modelling appropriate behaviour and supervising play (Odom et al., 1993, 1996). Alternatively, however, they sometimes create barriers by not supporting children with disabilities to engage in a wide and varied range of play activities (Ozen et al., 2013) or by limiting opportunities to make choices, take risks, embrace challenges, and make friends (Richardson 2002).

Educational professionals without appropriate levels of knowledge and sensitivity may also deny the opportunity for play through the educational policy that they deliver (Buchanon & Johnson, 2009; Richardson, 2002).

16.2.3 Barriers at Home

'Home' is a contested concept associated with a range of meanings and environments. Most importantly, 'home' is what each individual understands it to be. For children with disabilities, home may refer to the private family, but also to diverse care settings (e.g., hospitals or orphanages). Home may be a space supporting playfulness, when compared to other settings, particularly as the child ages (Law et al., 2007; Rigby & Gaik, 2007). Nevertheless, evidence suggests that barriers exist here.

Evidence of physical barriers include children with disabilities requiring assistance transferring between play spaces (e.g., up or down stairs), lack of space to manoeuvre wheelchairs, or so much space being taken up by assistive technologies and other equipment that accommodating visits from friends becomes difficult (Brotherson et al., 2008; Connors & Stalker 2003; Geisthardt et al., 2002). Additionally, attitudinal barriers manifest within home. Parents can be highly supportive of their child's play, but evidence suggests that some struggle to come to terms with their child's impairment and delay making physical adaptations to the home that would remove physical barriers to play (Lewis, 1987). Peers' attitudes may mean that children with disabilities are not always invited to friends' homes to play; equally, they may not be encouraged or supported to invite friends to come to their homes to play (Mundhenke et al., 2010; Sandberg et al., 2004). Parents' perceptions of risk may be important here: some parents have been found to restrict play in the home or not allow friends to visit for play due to perceptions of 'risk' (Connors & Stalker, 2003). Additionally, this may reflect concerns of parents regarding bullying and difficulties that non-disabled children may have knowing how to play with their children (Oates et al., 2011; Preece & Jordan, 2009). Barriers to play in the home may then reinforce barriers in other settings: research has shown that children with ASD, who have fewer playdates organised for them in the home, find engaging in play with peers in the school playground more difficult (Frankel et al., 2011).

16.2.4 Barriers in the Natural Environment

Identifying entirely natural settings in our world is challenging. There are few untouched wildernesses today (Cronon, 1996). Most natural environments that children encounter will be to some extent managed or modified by humans (Lester & Maudsley, 2007). Nevertheless, many authors agree that 'natural' spaces exhibit fewer elements of human design than 'built' environments. The value of play in the natural environment has been given increasing attention recently. Concerns about a 'couch potato' generation of children glued to electronic media (Hancox, 2004) and a 'bubble-wrap' generation of children whose parents are too anxious to let them play outside (Malone, 2007) are associated with increased valuing and promotion of play in nature (Louv, 2005).

Several studies have emphasised the benefits of playing in and with nature for children with and without disabilities (Blakesley et al., 2013; Pavey 2006; Kuo & Faber Taylor, 2004). As noted earlier, however, the primary focus of studies considering access to outdoor play for children with disabilities has been primarily on built environments such as playgrounds (e.g., Moore & Lynch, 2015; Webb, 2003). The right of access to nature for all children—a right referenced in the UNCRC—has often been forgotten (Anderson-Brolin, 2002). Whilst various reports (for organisations such as Play England and Barnados) highlight the importance of accessibility vis-a-vis, natural environments for children with disabilities and cite examples of good practice (Shackell et al., 2008; Lester & Maudsley, 2007), their overall message is that accessibility and inclusion are currently the exception rather than the rule.

Little research has been undertaken that explores barriers to play within natural environments for children with disabilities. Nevertheless, there is evidence of a range of barriers faced by all people with disabilities when seeking to access the natural environment, which would be worthy of further exploration vis-a-vis the experiences of children with disabilities, in particular. Barriers include insufficient information about physical accessibility, inadequate personal and private transport, inaccessible facilities, and staff attitudes at sites (Burns et al., 2008; Countryside Agency, 2005; Williams et al., 2004). Attitudes held by some professionals and parents can also be a significant barrier to 'nature play' for children with disabilities. For example, staff at outdoor recreation sites have been found to view outdoor, less-supervised activities to be 'too risky' for children with disabilities (Gleave, 2010). Similarly, Ludvigsen et al. (2005) found that some parents of children with disabilities, although initially positive about the idea of adventure play, perceived play sites to be 'unsafe'. Children with disabilities have indicated that such 'over-protection' limits opportunities for creativity, risk-taking, and physical challenge, all key factors in play (Andrews, 2012).

16.3 Discussion

This chapter considers the ways in which the social environment may limit the opportunities for play for children with disabilities, but is not an exhaustive consideration of this issue. We highlight, for example, the absence of consideration within the current research of socio-economic factors that may impact on play for children with disabilities. Economic barriers are likely to require further investigation, alongside wider environmental factors that may indirectly or directly affect access to play for these children—for example, the intersection of disability with other social and cultural factors relating to gender or ethnicity. The interaction of diverse socio-demographic characteristics deserves further attention.

Adults (teachers, parents, and other professionals) clearly have a key role in relation to facilitating play for children with disabilities. The tensions noted in educational settings and built environments between facilitating inclusion and limiting self-determination, as well as the barriers that may be created by the disabling attitudes of adults, require further research to identify strategies that can overcome these attitudes and balance adult facilitation with child-directed play.

In relation to unequal play opportunities for children with disabilities, the barriers created by impairments themselves must not be forgotten, but it is vitally important to recognise that any intervention at the individual level needs to be considered *in relation* to the environmental factors. Only by addressing disabling barriers external to the minds and bodies of individual children can we address the disablism, which disadvantages them, and remove obstacles to their right to play.

Finally, we suggest a framework for researching environmental barriers to play for children with disabilities. It is important to view the social environment encountered by children from the most immediate and personal through to the broadest social or societal. Various dimensions of a child's social environment might be examined, as follows (adapted from Brown, 2001):

- Accessibility: can children go where they would like to go? Are they fully included? Can they do what they would like to do?
- Resourcing: are their needs being met in ways that enable their play?
- Social support or enablement: are they welcomed and supported by those around them (peers and others)?
- Equality: are they treated equally compared with other children? Are they receiving equal opportunities for play?

The purpose of this list is not to rank different types of locations, but rather to understand the different types of interaction that individuals have with the environmental factors in given locations. It provides ideas about the types of intervention that might ensure that environmental factors become facilitators, not barriers to play for children with disabilities.

References

Anderson-Brolin, L. (2002). *The Rights of the Child and the Physical Environment - The UN Convention on the Rights of the Child and other Relevant International Agreements [report]*. Retrieved from: http://resourcecentre.savethechildren.se/sites/default/files/documents/2419.pdf.

Andrews, M. (2012). *Exploring Play for early Childhood Studies*. London, UK: Sage.

Atmakur, S. (2013). *Focus: Playgrounds of exclusion*. Retrieved from: http://www.unicef.org/sowc(2013)/focus_playgrounds_of_inclusion.html.

Barnes, C., & Mercer, G. (2010). *Exploring Disability: a Sociological Introduction* (2nd ed.). Cambridge, UK: Polity.

Barnett, E., & Casper, M. (2001). A definition of "social environment". [Letter to the editor]. *American Journal of Public Health*, 91, 465.

Barron, C., Beckett, A. E., Cannon-Jones, N., Coussens, M., Desoete, A., Fenney, D., Lynch, H., & Prellwitz, M. (*Forthcoming*). Barriers to Play and Recreation for Children with Disabilities. Berlin, D: De Gruyter.

Beckett, A. E., & Campbell, T. (2015). The social model of disability as an oppositional device. *Disability and Society*, 30, 270-283.

Bickenback, J. E. (2012). The International Classification of Functioning, Disability and Health and its relationship to disability studies. In N. Watson, A. Roulstone, & C. Thomas (Eds.), *Routledge Handbook of Disability Studies* (pp. 51-66). Abingdon, UK: Routledge.

Blakesley, D., Rickinson, M., & Dillon, J. (2013). *Engaging Children on the Autistic Spectrum with the Natural environment: Teacher insight study and evidence review* (Natural England Commissioned Report NECR 116). London, UK: Natural England.

Borsay, A. (1986). Personal Trouble or Public Issue? Towards a Model of Policy for People with Physical and Mental Disabilities. *Disability, Handicap and Society*, 1, 179-195.

Brotherson, M. J., Cook, C. C., Erwin, E. J., & Weigel, C. J. (2008). Understanding self-determination and families of young children with disabilities in home environments. *Journal of Early Intervention*, 31, 22-43.

Brown, S. C. (2001). Methodological Paradigms That Shape Disability Research. In G. L. Albrecht, K. D. Seelman, & M. Bury (Eds.), *Handbook of Disability Studies* (pp. 145-170). London, UK: Sage.

Buchanon, M., & Johnson, T. G. (2009). A Second look at play for Young Children with Disabilities. *American Journal of Play*, 2, 41-59.

Burns, N., Paterson, K., & Watson, N. (2008). *Exploring Disabled People's Perceptions and Use of Forest Recreation Goods, Facilities and Services in Scotland, England and Wales [report]*. Strathclyde Centre for Disability Research, UK. Retrieved from: http://www.forestry.gov.uk/pdf/SCDR_2008_Disabled_perceptions_and_woodland.pdf/$FILE/SCDR_2008_Disabled_perceptions_and_woodland.pdf.

Connors, C., & Stalker, K. (2003). *The Views and Experiences of Disabled Children and Their Siblings: A Positive Outlook*. London, UK: Jessica Kingsley Publishers.

Countryside Agency. (2005). *"WHAT ABOUT US?" Diversity Review evidence—part one. [report]*. Retrieved from: http://www.naturalengland.org.uk/ourwork/enjoying/outdoorsforall/diversityreview/publications/default.aspx.

Cronon, W. (1996). The trouble with wilderness: or, getting back to the wrong nature. *Environmental History*, 1, 7-28.

Dunn, K., & Moore, M. (2005). Developing accessible play space in the UK: a social model approach. *Children, Youth and Environments*, 15, 331-354.

Engel-Yeger, B., Jams, T., Anaby, D., & Law, M. (2009). Differences in patterns of participation between youths with cerebral palsy and typically developing peers. *American Journal of Occupational Therapy*, 63, 96-104.

Frankel, F., Gorospe, C., Chang, Y., & Sugar, C. (2011). Mothers' reports of play dates and observation of school playground behaviour of children having high-functioning autism spectrum disorders. *Journal of Child Psychology and Psychiatry*, 52, 571-579.

Geisthardt, C. L., Brotherson, M., Cook, & Christine, C. (2002). Friendships of Children with Disabilities in the Home Environment. *Education and Training in Mental Retardation and Developmental Disabilities*, 37, 235-52.

Gleave, J. (2010). *Making it Our Place: Community Views on Children's Play.* London, UK: Play England. Retrieved from: http://socialwelfare.bl.uk/subject-areas/services-client-groups/children-young-people/playengland/making10.aspx.

Goodley, D. (2014). *Dis/ability Studies—Theorising Disablism and Ableism*. Oxon: Routledge.

Goodley, D., & Runswick-Cole, C. (2010). Emancipating play: dis/abled children, development and deconstruction. *Disability and Society*, 25, 499-512.

Gustavsson, A., Tøssebro, J., & R. Traustadóttir (2005). Introduction: Approaches and perspectives in Nordic disability research. In A. Gustavsson, J. Sandvin, R. Traustadóttir, & J. Tøssebro (Eds.), *Resistance, Reflection and Change: Nordic Disability Research* (pp. 23-44). Lund, S: Student literature.

Hancox, B. (2005). Growing 'couch potatoes': television, computers and childhood obesity as a response to Gard (2004). *Children's Issues: Journal of the Children's Issues Centre*, 9, 32-36.

Hilton, C. L., Crouch, M. C., & Israel, H. (2008). Out-of-school participation patterns in children with high-functioning autism spectrum disorders. *American Journal of Occupational Therapy*, 62, 554-563.

Hurst, R. (2000). To revise or not to revise? *Disability and Society*, 15, 1083-1087.

Imms, C. (2008). Children with Cerebral Palsy Participate: A Review of the Literature. *Disability and Rehabilitation*, 30, 1867-1884.

Joseph, J., & Roberts, J.M. (2004) Introduction: realism, discourse and deconstruction. In: J. Joseph & J. M. Roberts (Eds.), *Realism, discourse and deconstruction* (pp.1-20). London, UK: Routledge.

Kuo, F., & Faber Taylor, A. (2004). A potential natural treatment for Attention-Deficit Hyperactivity disorder: evidence from a national study. *American Journal of Public Health*, 94, 1580-1586.

Law, M., Haight, M., Milroy, B., Williams, D., Stewart, D., & Rosenbaum, P. (1999). Environmental factors affecting the occupations of children with physical disabilities. *Journal of Occupational Science*, 6, 102-110.

Law, M. Petrenchik, T., King, G., & Hurley, P. (2007). Perceived environmental barriers to recreational, community, and school participation for children and youth with physical disabilities. *Archives of Physical Medicine and Rehabilitation*, 88, 1636-1642.

Lester, S., & Maudsley, M. (2007). *Play naturally: a review of children's natural play*. London, UK: National Children's Bureau and Play England.

Lewis, B. (1987). How are families managing at home? Architectural barriers in households of children with special needs- an issue ignored by health professional. *Children's Environments Quarterly*, 4, 36-41.

Louv, R. (2005). *Last Child in the Woods: Saving our Children from Nature-Deficit Disorder*. London, UK: Atlantic Books.

Ludvigsen, A., Creegan, C., & Mills, H. (2005). *Let's Play Together: Play and Inclusion. Evaluation of Better Play Round Three [report]*. Retrieved from: www.barnardos.org.uk/lets_play_together_report.pdf.

Malone, K. (2007). The bubble-wrap generation: children growing up in walled gardens. *Environmental Education Research*, 13, 513-527.

McLaughlin, J. (2006). Conceptualising Intensive Caring Activities: the Changing Lives of Families with Young Disabled Children. *Sociological Research Online*, 11.

Moore, A., & Lynch, H. (2015). Accessibility and usability of playground environments for children under 12: A scoping review. *Scandinavian Journal of Occupational Therapy*, 22, 331-334.

Moyles, J. (2013). *Play and Early Years* [webpage]. Retrieved from: http://www.playwales.org.

Mundhenke, L., Hermansson, L., & Nattterland, B. (2010). Experiences of Swedish children with disabilities: activities and social support in daily life. *Scandinavian Journal of Occupational Therapy*, 17, 130-139.

Nilsen, R. D., & Rogers, B. (2005). "That's not a good idea, mom": Negotiating children's subjectivity while constructing 'home' as a research site. *Children's Geographies*, 3, 345-362.

Oates, A., Bebbington, A., Bourke, J., Girdler, S., & Leonard, H. (2011). Leisure participation for school-aged children with Down syndrome. *Disability and Rehabilitation*, 33, 1880-1889.
Odom, S. L., Peck, C. A., Hanson, M., Beckman, P. J., Kaiser, A. P., Lieber, J., ... & Schwartz, I. S. (1996). Inclusion at the preschool level: An ecological systems analysis. *Social Policy: Society for Research on Child Development*, 10, 18-30.
Oliver, M. (1990). *The Politics of Disablement.* Basingstoke, UK: The Macmillan Press Ltd.
Oliver, M., & Barnes, C. (2011) *The New Politics of Disablement.* Tavistock, UK: Palgrave.
Ozen, A., Ergonekon, Y., Ulke-Kurkcuoglu, B., & Genç, D. (2013). Opinions of special education teachers about activity-based intervention. *H.U. Journal of Education*, 44, 262-274.
Pavey, B. (2005). *The Forest School and Inclusion: a Project evaluation [report].* University of Leeds. Retrieved from: http://www.leeds.ac.uk/educol/documents/161165.doc.
Preece, D., & Jordan, R. (2010) Obtaining the views of children and young people with autism spectrum disorders about their experience of daily life and social care support. *British Journal of Learning Disabilities*, 38, 1354-4187.
Prellwitz, M. (2007). Playground accessibility and usability for children with disabilities. PhD thesis: Lulea University of Technology, Sweden.
Prellwitz, M., & Skar, L. (2007). Usability of playgrounds for children with different abilities. *Occupational Therapy International*, 14, 144-155.
Prellwitz, M. & Tamm, M. (1999). Attitudes of key persons to accessibility problems in playgrounds for children with restricted mobility: A study in a medium-sized municipality in northern Sweden. *Scandinavian Journal of Occupational Therapy*, 6, 166-173.
Priestley, M. (1998). Childhood disability and disabled childhoods. Agendas for research. *Childhood*, 5, 207-223.
Richardson, P. K. (2002). The School as Social Context: Social Interaction. Patterns of Children with Physical Disabilities. *American Journal of Occupational Therapy*, 56, 296–304.
Rigby, P., & Gaik, S. (2007). Stability of Playfulness Across Environmental Settings. A Pilot Study. *Physical and Occupational Therapy in Paediatrics*, 27, 27-43.
Rimmer, J. H., Riley B., Wang, E., Rauworth, A., & Jurkowski, J. (2004). Physical activity participation among persons with disabilities: barriers and facilitators. *American Journal of Preventive Medicine*, 26, 419-25.
Sandberg, A., Bjorck-Akesson, E., & Granlund, M. (2004). Play in retrospection: play experiences from childhood in adults with visual disability, motor disability and Asperger syndrome. *Scandinavian Journal of Disability Research*, 6, 111-130.
Santer, J., Griffiths, C., & Goodall, D. (2007). *Free Play in Early Childhood [report].* London, UK. Play England. Retrieved from: http://www.playengland.org.uk/media/120426/free-play-in-early-childhood.pdf.
Sense (2016). *Making the case for play. Findings of the Sense Public Inquiry into Access to Play Opportunities for Disabled Children with Multiple Needs [report].* London, UK: Sense. Retrieved from https://www.sense.org.uk/sites/default/files/the-case-for-play-report.pdf.
Shackell, A., Butler, N., Doyle, P., & Ball, D. (2008). *Design for Play: A Guide to Creating Successful Play Spaces [report].* Play England. Retrieved from http://www.playengland.org.uk/resources/design-for-play.aspx.
Shakespeare, T. (2014). *Disability rights and wrongs revisited.* Abingdon, UK: Routledge.
Spencer-Cavaliere, N., & Watkinson, E. J. (2010). Inclusion understood from the perspectives of children with disability. *Adapted Physical Activity Quarterly*, 27, 275-93.
Sutton-Smith, B. 1997. *The Ambiguity of Play.* Cambridge, MA: Harvard University Press.
Taub, D. E., & Greer, K. R. (2000). Physical Activity as a Normalizing Experience for School-Age Children with Physical Disabilities. Implications for Legitimation of Social Identity and Enhancement of Social Ties. *Sport and Social Issues*, 24, 395-414.

Thomas, C. (2004). Developing the Social Relational in the Social Model of Disability: a theoretical agenda. In: C. Barnes, & G. Mercer (Eds.), *Implementing the Social Model of Disability: Theory and Research* (pp. 32-47). Leeds, UK: Disability Press.
United Nations (2007). *Convention on the Rights of Persons with Disabilities*. Retrieved from: http://www.un.org/disabilities/convention/conventionfull.shtml.
UNCRC Committee on the Rights of the Child (2016). *Concluding Observations on the Fifth Periodic Report of the United Kingdom of Great Britain and Northern Ireland*. DRAFT. Retrieved from: tbinternet.ohchr.org/Treaties/CRC/.../GBR/INT_CRC_IFN_GBR_21049_E.pdf.
Union of the Physically Impaired Against Segregation, UPIAS (1975). *Fundamental Principles of Disability*. [Statement]. Retrieved from: http://www.disabilityarchive.leeds.ac.uk/authors_list.asp?AuthorID=174&author_name=UPIAS.
Webb, R. (2003). *Public Play Provision for Children with Disabilities*. Sugradh, IRL: NDA
World Health Organisation (2011). *World Report on Disability*. Retrieved from: http://www.who.int/disabilities/world_report/2011/en/.
World Health Organisation (2001). *International Classification of Functioning Disability and Health*. Geneva, CH: WHO.
Williams, R., Vogelsong, H., Green, G., & Cordell, K. (2004). Outdoor Recreation Participation of People with Mobility Disabilities: "Selected Results of the National Survey of Recreation and the Environment. *Journal of Park and Recreation Administration*, 22, 85-101.
Woolley, H. (2013). Now Being Social: The Barrier of Designing Outdoor Play Spaces for Disabled Children. *Children and Society*, 27, 448-458.

Serenella Besio, Daniela Bulgarelli,
and Vaska Stancheva-Popkostadinova

Conclusion

This book is the first systematisation of the theme of play for children with disabilities, within the specific frame of 'play for the sake of play'.

It was meant to reflect the state of the art about play and children with disabilities up to 2015, to become a useful tool for professionals and researchers in all the related fields, and mainly to establish a point of reference for building up new knowledge on this theme, trying to address the collective scientific discussion towards this new framework.

The International Classification of Functioning, Disability and Health is undoubtedly the most authoritative framing of impairment and disability, describing the human functioning as a complex result of a system of interrelations between the persons' body, the environment in which they live, the personal determinants, and the continuous necessary tension towards activity and participation.

This book wants to lay the groundwork for an overall exploration of the theme of play for children with disabilities. After an overview of children's play in the literature, in search of firm and shared points of reference, it proposes—through comparison with the existing proposals—its two main classifications, the first concerning the types of play that occur along the child's development (variously intertwined) and the second relating to the types of disabilities that will be included in the study.

These introductory parts lead to discuss, in more depth, the characteristics that play can assume for children with various types of impairments, according to the studies published at the international level. Then, the text completes the background, thanks to some final chapters that explore the contribution of some disciplines deeply involved in the theme—occupational therapy, special education, early intervention—propose a professional perspective on the assessment and choice of toys, and finally, deal with the main environmental factors that can create barriers to the full deployment of the child's play.

The chapters' authors—coming from various countries and different disciplines—were then given a not easy task, mainly due to the fact that they have been requested to treat the theme according to the particular constraints given by the described framework.

The most important challenges they had to face were: a) the existing studies usually treat the concept of play as a well-known and universal one, without adopting a specific definition; b) in particular, the awareness about the difference between play and play-like activities is not represented at all in the literature of play for children with disabilities; and c) a variety of proliferating types of play are presented and explored, but not rooted on precise descriptions, and this contributes to create misconceptions, thus lowering the possibility to open plain debates at a scientific level, to compare the results of different experimentations, to build new knowledge and new professional practice on the possible new shared findings.

But the main novelty of this text is to stress the concept of 'play for the sake of play' and to introduce a specific attention to this interpretation of play in the case of children with disabilities.

In fact, misconceptions of play create some overlapping in the literature between the two constructs of 'play for the sake of play' and 'play-like activities': and this is even more true when it comes to the case of children with disabilities, where play is almost uniquely considered as a technique to obtain educational improvements or as a clinical evidence to assess the child's development.

It is only the case to remind here that this creates, in turn, additional theoretical problems, where it happens that 'play for the sake of play' starts to be described in the literature as 'free play', thus loosing its specific and multifaceted characteristics at an alarming extent, which cannot be confused in a sole shapeless pot. When play is free—that means it is made only for the sake of itself—it might belong to very different types and these ones should be very carefully explored.

Moreover, it is exactly play for the sake of play that is a right for all children and should be claimed for, as testified by the most important international conventions, and should be guaranteed to all children, including those who have some impairments: play activities should be then accessible and inclusive with respect to contexts, tools (toys, playgrounds, and other instruments), support methodologies (if they occur within educational contexts), and relationships. And, this requires a radical change in the societal attitudes and scientific approaches, a specific training for educational, health, and social professionals, but also new directions in the overall policies, including the investment of economic resources.

Play in children with disabilities is a new scientific topic and this book reflects this novelty. It still suffers from some heterogeneity, because a comprehensive theoretical framework is far to be reached in the general literature and it is the first product of a brand-new scientific community, which is at the same time, international and interdisciplinary, thus representing different experiences and cultural climates as well as different scientific fields, which needs to find the most productive way to encounter and create their own language and establish their fundamentals.

As editors of this publication and members of the network 'LUDI—Play for Children with Disabilities', we consider this as a first step of the Action's contribution to the scientific community. Further products will come, developed by the other Working Groups in which the Action is built upon, and the overall LUDI framework will result, at the end, as a sort of construction made of Lego bricks that fit perfectly one with the other to create the final perfect shape.

Many aspects should be further deepened, and we would like to remark here the most important ones.

- The voice of children with disabilities and of their parents should be carefully collected and included, to the point of questioning the findings already reached.

- The role, the type, the characteristics of tools and of technologies should be investigated with respect to the various types of play described, and this will hopefully bring many important suggestions to the field of technology development as well as to the professional practice.
- The various possible roles that adults can assume within and in favour of the children's play activities will be more explored in the next studies: they can be as competent play companions, can use suitable methods for assessment, and can act as supporters of this new scientific topic.
- The inclusive aspects of play should be deeply examined and treated as the only, unavoidable, context to express play for the sake of play: this means to lead the way towards big changes, in attitudes, procedures, and methodologies of intervention; societies at large should become more accessible, more flexible, more open to diversity.

Finally, a natural outcome of the LUDI's work will be to clearly locate play as one of the areas to establish and measure the Quality of Life (QoL) in children with disabilities.

QoL is related to the possibility of being autonomous and to the possibility of inclusively taking part to everyday-life contexts. In children's life, play is crucial to actively experience autonomy and inclusiveness: during play, children can take autonomous decisions and freely organise their activities, they can experience the social dimension of life while interacting with other play companions, peers, or adults.

But autonomy might be often reduced or even precluded to children with disabilities: whenever their functional limitations face environmental factors, which prevent them from making the right and effective experiences, they cannot access play activities in a fruitful and proactive way. In terms of ICF, they can show a disability, due to the physical impairments and/or to wrong, excluding, not usable or not accessible environmental factors: the human field—methods, relationships, social attitudes, and so on—and in the concrete world—objects, architecture, structures, and so on—can, in fact, create barriers that prevent them from participation.

Building up research, knowledge, and societal attention around the topic of play in children with disabilities is one of the fundamental steps towards the possibility to support every child's QoL.

Bei Fragen zur Produktsicherheit wenden Sie sich bitte an:
If you have any questions regarding product safety,
please contact:

Walter de Gruyter GmbH
Genthiner Straße 13
10785 Berlin
productsafety@degruyterbrill.com